IARC MONOGRAPHS
ON THE
EVALUATION OF THE CARCINOGENIC RISK
OF CHEMICALS TO MAN:

Cadmium, Nickel, Some Epoxides, Miscellaneous Industrial Chemicals and General Considerations on Volatile Anaesthetics

Volume 11

This publication represents the views of two
IARC Working Groups on the
Evaluation of the Carcinogenic Risk of Chemicals to Man
which met in Lyon,
9-11 December 1975 and 3-9 February 1976

IARC WORKING GROUP ON THE EVALUATION OF THE CARCINOGENIC RISK OF CHEMICALS
TO MAN: CADMIUM AND NICKEL*

Lyon, 9-11 December 1975

Members[1]

Dr U.H. Ehling, Gesellschaft für Strahlen- und Umweltforschung MBH München, Institut für Biologie, Abteilung für Genetik, Ingolstädter Landstrasse 1, Post Oberschleissheim, D-8042 Neuherberg, FRG

Dr E. Pedersen, Director, The Cancer Registry of Norway, Institute for Epidemiological Research, The Norwegian Radium Hospital, Oslo 3, Norway (*Vice-Chairman*)

Dr M. Piscator, The Karolinska Institute, Department of Environmental Hygiene, S-104 01 Stockholm 60, Sweden

Dr U. Saffiotti, Associate Director for Carcinogenesis, Division of Cancer Cause and Prevention, National Cancer Institute, Bethesda, Maryland 20014, USA

Dr R. Saracci[2], Chief, Biostatistics and Clinical Epidemiology Section, CNR Laboratory for Clinical Physiology, University of Pisa, Via Savi 8, 56100 Pisa, Italy

Professor H.-W. Schlipköter, Direktor des Medizinischen Instituts für Lufthygiene und Silikoseforschung und des Instituts für Hygiene der Universität Düsseldorf, Gurlittstrasse 53, D-4 Düsseldorf, FRG

Professor I.J. Selikoff, Mount Sinai School of Medicine of the City University of New York, Department of Community Medicine, Fifth Avenue and 100th Street, New York, NY 10029, USA

Dr F.W. Sunderman, Jr, Professor and Head, Department of Laboratory Medicine, University of Connecticut School of Medicine, Box G, Farmington, Connecticut 06032, USA

---

*Asbestos was also considered by this Working Group, but a decision concerning the publication of the monograph has not yet been taken.

[1]Unable to attend: Dr V.B. Okulov, Petrov Research Institute of Oncology, 68 Leningradskaya Street, Pesochny-2, Leningrad 188646, USSR

[2]Present address: Unit of Epidemiology and Biostatistics, International Agency for Research on Cancer, 150 Cours Albert Thomas, 69372 Lyon Cédex 2, France

Dr J.C. Wagner, Medical Research Council Pneumoconiosis Unit, Llandough Hospital, Penarth, Glamorgan CF6 lXW, South Wales, UK

Dr J.K. Wagoner, Director, Division of Field Studies and Clinical Investigation, National Institute of Occupational Safety and Health, US Post Office and Court House, 5th and Main Streets, Cincinnati, Ohio 45202, USA (*Chairman*)

Invited Guests

Dr A. Annoni, Occupational Safety and Health Branch, International Labour Office, CH-1211 Geneva 22, Switzerland

Dr J. Bignon, Clinique de Pneumo-Phtisiologie, Hôpital Laennec, 42 rue de Sèvres, 75007 Paris, France

Dr P. Westerholm, National Board of Occupational Safety and Health, Wennerbergsgatan 10, 10026 Stockholm 34, Sweden

Secretariat

Dr C. Agthe, Unit of Chemical Carcinogenesis (*Secretary*)

Dr N. Day, Unit of Epidemiology and Biostatistics

Dr R.A. Lemen, Chief, Biometry Branch of Field Studies and Clinical Investigation, National Institute of Occupational Safety & Health, US Post Office and Court House, 5th and Main Streets, Cincinnati, Ohio 45202, USA (*Temporary Advisor*)

Dr R. Maclennan, Unit of Epidemiology and Biostatistics

Dr B. Marschall, Medical Officer, Occupational Health, WHO, Geneva

Mrs C. Partensky, Unit of Chemical Carcinogenesis

Mrs I. Peterschmitt, Unit of Chemical Carcinogenesis, Geneva

Dr L. Tomatis, Chief, Unit of Chemical Carcinogenesis

Mr E.A. Walker, Unit of Environmental Carcinogens

Mrs E. Ward, Montignac, France (*Editor*)

Mr J.D. Wilbourn, Unit of Chemical Carcinogenesis

IARC WORKING GROUP ON THE EVALUATION OF THE CARCINOGENIC RISK OF CHEMICALS
TO MAN: SOME EPOXIDES, MISCELLANEOUS INDUSTRIAL CHEMICALS AND
GENERAL CONSIDERATIONS ON VOLATILE ANAESTHETICS

Lyon, 3-9 February 1976

Members

Dr R.K. Boutwell, Professor of Oncology, McArdle Laboratory for Cancer Research, University of Wisconsin, Medical Center, Madison, Wisconsin 53706, USA (*Vice-Chairman*)

Professor E. Boyland, Institute of Occupational Health, London School of Hygiene and Tropical Medicine, Keppel Street, London WC1E 7HT, UK (*Chairman*)

Dr T.H. Corbett, Clinical Investigator, Research Service, US Veterans Administration Hospital, Ann Arbor, Michigan 48105, USA

Dr L. Fishbein, Assistant to the Director for Environmental Surveillance, National Center for Toxicological Research, Jefferson, Arkansas 72079, USA

Dr D.E. Hathway, Senior Research Scientist, Central Toxicology Laboratory, Imperial Chemical Industries Ltd, Alderley Park, Nr Macclesfield, Cheshire SK10 4TJ, UK

Professor N. Loprieno, Director, CNR Laboratory of Mutagenesis and Differentiation, Via Cisanello 147/B, 56100 Pisa, Italy

Professor F. Oesch, Head, Section on Biochemical Pharmacology, Johannes Gutenberg-Universität Mainz, Pharmakologisches Institut, Obere Zahlbacher Strasse 67, D-6500 Mainz, FRG

Dr G. Rudali, Directeur de Recherches, Fondation Curie - Institut du Radium, Section de Biologie, 26 rue d'Ulm, 75231 Paris Cédex 05, France

Dr R. Saracci[1], Chief, Biostatistics & Clinical Epidemiology Section, CNR Laboratory for Clinical Physiology, University of Pisa, Via Savi 8, 56100 Pisa, Italy

Dr B. Teichmann, Akademie der Wissenschaften der DDR, Zentralinstitut für Krebsforschung, Lindenberger Weg 80, 1115 Berlin-Buch, GDR

Professor R. Truhaut, Directeur, Centre de recherches toxicologiques, Faculté des Sciences pharmaceutiques et biologiques de l'Université René Descartes, 4 Avenue de l'Observatoire, 75006 Paris, France

---

[1]Present address: Unit of Epidemiology and Biostatistics, International Agency for Research on Cancer, 150 Cours Albert Thomas, 69372 Lyon Cédex 2, France

Dr V.S. Turusov, Cancer Research Center, USSR Academy of Medical Sciences, Karshirskoye Shosse 6, Moscow 115478, USSR

Dr B.L. Van Duuren, Professor of Environmental Medicine, New York University Medical Center, Institute of Environmental Medicine, 550 First Avenue, New York, NY 10016, USA

Dr J.S. Wassom, Director, Environmental Mutagen Information Center, Oak Ridge National Laboratory, PO Box Y, Oak Ridge, Tennessee 37830, USA

Invited Guests[1]

Dr A. Annoni, Occupational Safety & Health Branch, International Labour Office, CH-1211 Geneva 22, Switzerland

Dr J.J. Clary, Manager, Toxicology, E.I. Du Pont de Nemours & Co., Inc., Central Research & Development Department, Haskell Laboratory for Toxicology and Industrial Medicine, Wilmington, Delaware 19898, USA

Dr K.E. McCaleb, Director, Chemical-Environmental Program, Chemical Industries Center, Stanford Research Institute, Menlo Park, California 94025, USA (*Rapporteur sections 2.1 and 2.2*)

Dr L. Rinzema, Dow Chemical Europe S.A., CH-8810 Horgen, Switzerland

Dr P. Westerholm, Deputy Medical Director, National Board of Occupational Safety and Health, Medical Department, Wennerbergsgatan 10, 10026 Stockholm 34, Sweden

Secretariat

    Dr C. Agthe, Unit of Chemical Carcinogenesis (*Secretary*)

    Dr H. Bartsch, Unit of Chemical Carcinogenesis (*Rapporteur section 3.1*)

    Dr L. Griciute, Chief, Unit of Environmental Carcinogens

    Dr B. Marschall, Occupational Health Unit, WHO, Geneva

    Dr R. Montesano, Unit of Chemical Carcinogenesis (*Rapporteur section 3.1*)

    Mrs C. Partensky, Unit of Chemical Carcinogenesis (*Technical editor*)

    Mrs I. Peterschmitt, Unit of Chemical Carcinogenesis, Geneva (*Bibliographic researcher*)

    Dr V. Ponomarkov, Unit of Chemical Carcinogenesis

    Dr L. Tomatis, Chief, Unit of Chemical Carcinogenesis (*Head of the Programme*)

---

[1]Unable to attend: Dr M. Sharratt, Senior Medical Officer, Department of Health & Social Security, Alexander Fleming House, Elephant and Castle, London SE1 6BY, UK

Mr E.A. Walker, Unit of Environmental Carcinogens (*Rapporteur sections 1 and 2.3*)

Mrs E. Ward, Montignac, France (*Editor*)

Mr J.D. Wilbourn, Unit of Chemical Carcinogenesis (*Co-secretary*)

Note to the reader

Every effort is made to present the monographs as accurately as possible without unduly delaying their publication. Nevertheless, mistakes have occurred and are still likely to occur. In the interest of all users of these monographs, readers are requested to communicate any errors observed to the Unit of Chemical Carcinogenesis of the International Agency for Research on Cancer, Lyon, France, in order that these can be included in corrigenda which will appear in subsequent volumes.

As stated in the preamble, great efforts are made to cover the whole literature, but some studies may have been inadvertently overlooked. Since the monographs are not intended to be a review of the literature and contain only data considered relevant by the Working Group, it is not possible for the reader to determine whether a certain study was considered or not. However, research workers who are aware of important published data which may change the evaluation are requested to make them available to the above-mentioned address, in order that they can be considered for a possible re-evaluation by a future Working Group.

CONTENTS

BACKGROUND AND PURPOSE OF THE IARC PROGRAMME ON THE EVALUATION
  OF THE CARCINOGENIC RISK OF CHEMICALS TO MAN 13

SCOPE OF THE MONOGRAPHS 13

MECHANISM FOR PRODUCING THE MONOGRAPHS 14

    Priority for the preparation of monographs 14
    Data on which the evaluation is based 14
    The Working Group 15

GENERAL PRINCIPLES FOR THE EVALUATION 15

    Terminology 15
    Response to carcinogens 16
    Purity of the compounds tested 16
    Qualitative aspects 16
    Quantitative aspects 17
    Animal data in relation to the evaluation of risk to man 17
    Evidence of human carcinogenicity 17

EXPLANATORY NOTES ON THE MONOGRAPHS 18

GENERAL REMARKS ON THE SUBSTANCES CONSIDERED 28

THE MONOGRAPHS

    Cadmium and cadmium compounds 39

    Nickel and nickel compounds 75

    Epoxides:

        Diepoxybutane 115
        Diglycidyl resorcinol ether 125
        Epichlorohydrin 131
        1-Epoxyethyl-3,4-epoxycyclohexane 141
        3,4-Epoxy-6-methylcyclohexylmethyl-3,4-epoxy-6-
            methylcyclohexane carboxylate 147
        cis-9,10-Epoxystearic acid 153
        Ethylene oxide 157

Fusarenon-X	169
Glycidaldehyde	175
Glycidyl oleate	183
Glycidyl stearate	187
Propylene oxide	191
Styrene oxide	201
Triethylene glycol diglycidyl ether	209

Miscellaneous industrial chemicals:

Benzyl chloride	217
β-Butyrolactone	225
γ-Butyrolactone	231
Dinitrosopentamethylenetetramine	241
1,4-Dioxane	247
Ethylene sulphide	257
Trichloroethylene	263
4-Vinylcyclohexene	277

General considerations on volatile anaesthetics	285
SUPPLEMENTARY CORRIGENDA TO VOLUMES 1-10	295
CUMULATIVE INDEX TO MONOGRAPHS	297

BACKGROUND AND PURPOSE OF THE IARC PROGRAMME ON THE EVALUATION OF THE CARCINOGENIC RISK OF CHEMICALS TO MAN

The International Agency for Research on Cancer (IARC) initiated in 1971 a programme on the evaluation of the carcinogenic risk of chemicals to man. This programme was supported by a Resolution of the Governing Council at its Ninth Session concerning the role of IARC in providing government authorities with expert, independent scientific opinion on environmental carcinogenesis. As one means to this end, the Governing Council recommended that IARC should continue to prepare monographs on the carcinogenic risk of individual chemicals to man.

In view of the importance of this programme and in order to expedite the production of monographs, the National Cancer Institute of the United States has provided IARC with additional funds for this purpose.

The objective of this programme is to elaborate and publish in the form of monographs a critical review of carcinogenicity and related data in the light of the present state of knowledge, with the final aim of evaluating the data in terms of possible human risk, and at the same time to indicate where additional research efforts are needed.

SCOPE OF THE MONOGRAPHS

The monographs summarize the evidence for the carcinogenicity of individual chemicals and other relevant information. The data are compiled, reviewed and evaluated by a Working Group of experts. No recommendations are given concerning preventive measures or legislation, since these matters depend on risk-benefit evaluation, which seems best made by individual governments and/or international agencies such as WHO and ILO.

Since 1971, when the programme was started, ten volumes have been published[1-10].

As new data on chemicals for which monographs have already been written and new principles for evaluation become available, re-evaluations will be made at future meetings, and revised monographs will be published as necessary. The monographs are distributed to international and governmental agencies and will be available to industries and scientists dealing with these chemicals. They also form the basis of advice from IARC on carcinogenesis from these substances.

MECHANISM FOR PRODUCING THE MONOGRAPHS

As a first step, a list of chemicals for possible consideration by the Working Group is established. IARC then collects pertinent references regarding physico-chemical characteristics, production and use*, occurrence and analysis, and biological data** on these compounds. The material is summarized by an expert consultant or an IARC staff member, who prepares the first draft, which in some cases is sent to another expert for comments. The drafts are circulated to all members of the Working Group about one month before the meeting. During the meeting further additions to and deletions from the data are agreed upon, and a final version of comments and evaluation on each compound is adopted.

Priority for the Preparation of Monographs

Priority is given mainly to chemicals belonging to groups for which at least some suggestion of carcinogenicity exists from observations in animals and/or man and for which there is evidence of human exposure. However, neither human exposure nor potential carcinogenicity can be judged until all the relevant data have been collected and examined in detail; thus, *the inclusion of a particular compound in a volume does not necessarily mean that the substance is considered to be carcinogenic. Equally, the fact that a substance has not yet been considered does not imply that it is without carcinogenic hazard.*

Data on which the Evaluation is Based

With regard to the biological data, only published articles and papers already accepted for publication are reviewed. Every effort is made to

---

*Data provided by Chemical Information Services, Stanford Research Institute, Menlo Park, California, USA

**In the collection of original data reference was made to the publications 'Survey of compounds which have been tested for carcinogenic activity'[11-16].

cover the whole literature, but some studies may have been inadvertently overlooked. The monographs are not intended to be a full review of the literature, and they contain only data considered relevant by the Working Group. Research workers who are aware of important data (published or accepted for publication) which may influence the evaluation are invited to make them available to the Unit of Chemical Carcinogenesis of the International Agency for Research on Cancer, Lyon, France.

The Working Group

The tasks of the Working Group are five-fold: (1) to verify that as far as feasible all data have been collected; (2) to select the data relevant for the evaluation; (3) to determine whether the data, as summarized, will enable the reader to follow the reasoning of the committee; (4) to judge the significance of results of experimental and epidemiological studies; and (5) to make an evaluation.

The members of the Working Group who participated in the consideration of particular substances are listed at the beginning of each publication. The members serve in their individual capacities as scientists and not as representatives of their governments or of any organization with which they are affiliated.

GENERAL PRINCIPLES FOR THE EVALUATION

The general principles for the evaluation which are listed below were elaborated by previous Working Groups and were also applied to the substances listed in this volume.

Terminology

The term 'chemical carcinogenesis' in its widely accepted sense is used to indicate the induction or enhancement of neoplasia by chemicals. It is recognized that, in the strict etymological sense, this term means the induction of cancer; however, common usage has led to its employment to denote the induction of various types of neoplasms. The terms 'tumourigen', 'oncogen' and 'blastomogen' have all been used synonymously with 'carcinogen', although occasionally 'tumourigen' has been used specifically to denote the induction of benign tumours.

Response to Carcinogens

For present purposes, in general, no distinction is made between the induction of tumours and the enhancement of tumour incidence, although it is noted that there may be fundamental differences in mechanisms that will eventually be elucidated.

The response in experimental animals to a carcinogen may take several forms:

(1) a significant increase in the incidence of one or more of the same types of neoplasms as found in control animals;

(2) the occurrence of types of neoplasms not observed in control animals;

(3) a decreased latent period for the production of neoplasms as compared with that in control animals.

Purity of the Compounds Tested

In any evaluation of biological data with respect to a possible carcinogenic risk, particular attention must be paid to the purity of the chemicals tested and to their stability under conditions of storage or administration. Information on purity and stability is given, when available, in the monographs.

Qualitative Aspects

The qualitative nature of neoplasia has been much discussed. In many instances, both benign and malignant tumours are induced by chemical carcinogens. There are so far few recorded instances in which only benign tumours are induced by chemicals that have been studied extensively. Their occurrence in experimental systems has been taken to indicate the possibility of an increased risk of malignant tumours also.

In experimental carcinogenesis, the type of cancer seen can be the same as that recorded in human studies (e.g., bladder cancer in man, monkeys, dogs and hamsters after administration of 2-naphthylamine). In other instances, however, a chemical can induce other types of neoplasms at different sites in various species (e.g., benzidine induces hepatic carcinoma in the rat, but bladder carcinoma in man).

Quantitative Aspects

Dose-response studies are important in the evaluation of human and animal carcinogenesis. The confidence with which a carcinogenic effect can be established is strengthened by the observation of an increasing incidence of neoplasms with increasing exposure. Such studies are the only ones on which a minimal effective dose can be established. The determination of such a dose allows a comparison with reliable data on human exposure.

Comparison of potency between compounds can only be made if and when substances have been tested simultaneously.

Animal Data in Relation to the Evaluation of Risk to Man

At the present time no attempt can be made to interpret the animal data directly in terms of human risk since no objective criteria are available to do so. The critical assessment of the validity of the animal data given in these monographs is intended to assist national and/or international authorities in making decisions concerning preventive measures or legislation. In this connection attention is drawn to WHO recommendations in relation to food additives[17], drugs[18] and occupational carcinogens[19].

Evidence of Human Carcinogenicity

Evaluation of the carcinogenic risk to man of suspected environmental agents rests on purely observational studies. Such studies require sufficient variation in the levels of human exposure to allow a meaningful relationship between cancer incidence and exposure to a given chemical to be established. Difficulties in isolating the effects of individual agents arise, however, since populations are exposed to multiple carcinogens.

The initial suggestion of a relationship between an agent and disease often comes from case reports of patients who have had similar exposures. Variations and time trends in regional or national cancer incidence, or their correlation with regional or national 'exposure' levels, may also provide valuable insights. Such observations by themselves, however, cannot in most circumstances be regarded as conclusive evidence of carcinogenicity. The most satisfactory epidemiological method is to compare the cancer risk (adjusted for age, sex and other confounding variables) among groups or cohorts, or among individuals exposed to various levels of the agent in question, and among control groups not so exposed. Ideally this is accomplished directly, by following such groups forward in time (prospectively) to determine time relationships, dose-response relationships and other aspects of cancer induction. Large cohorts and long observation periods are required to provide sufficient cases for a statistically valid comparison.

An alternative to prospective investigation is to assemble cohorts from past records and to evaluate their subsequent morbidity or mortality by means of medical histories and death certificates. Such occupational carcinogens as nickel, β-naphthylamine, asbestos and benzidine have been confirmed by this method. Another method is to compare the past exposures of a defined group of cancer cases with those of control cases from the hospital or general population. This does not provide an absolute measure of carcinogenic risk but can indicate the relative risks associated with different levels of exposure. The indirect means (e.g., interviews or tissue residues) used to measure exposures which may have commenced many years before can constitute a major source of error. Nevertheless such case-control studies can often isolate one factor from several suspected agents. The carcinogenic effect of this substance could then be confirmed by cohort studies.

EXPLANATORY NOTES ON THE MONOGRAPHS

In sections 1, 2 and 3 of each monograph, except for minor remarks, the data are recorded as given by the author, whereas the comments by the Working Group are given in section 4, headed 'Comments on Data Reported and Evaluation'.

Chemical and Physical Data (section 1)

The Chemical Abstracts Registry Serial Number and the latest Chemical Abstracts Name are recorded in this section, together with other synonyms and trade names.

Chemical and physical properties include, in particular, data that might be relevant to carcinogenicity (for example, lipid solubility) and those that concern identification. Where applicable, data on solubility, volatility and stability are indicated. Data for which no reference is given are usually taken from standard reference books such as the *Merck Index*[20] or the *Handbook of Chemistry and Physics*[21]. All chemical data in this section refer to the pure substance, unless otherwise specified.

Production, Use, Occurrence and Analysis (section 2)

The ultimate purpose of this section is to give an idea of the extent of possible human exposure, and therefore data on production, use and occurrence are given when available. With regard to these data, IARC has collaborated with the Stanford Research Institute, USA, with the support of the National Cancer Institute of the USA, in order to obtain production figures of chemicals and their patterns of use.

The United States, Europe and Japan are reasonably representative industrialized areas of the world, and if data on production or use are available from these countries they are reported. It should *not*, however, be inferred that these nations are the sole sources or even the major sources of any individual chemical.

Production data are obtained from both governmental and trade publications in the three geographic areas. Information on use and occurrence is obtained by a comprehensive review of published data, complemented by direct contact with manufacturers of the chemicals in question.

Since cancer is a delayed toxic effect, past use and production data are also of importance. With respect to past and present use and production, regulatory actions in some countries are mentioned as examples only. Statements concerning regulations may not reflect the most recent situation, since such legislation is in a constant state of change; nor should it be taken to imply that other countries do not have similar regulations. In the cases of drugs, mention of the therapeutic uses of such chemicals does not necessarily represent presently accepted therapeutic indications, nor does it imply judgement as to their clinical efficacy.

It is hoped that in future revisions of these monographs, more information on production and use can be made available to IARC from other countries.

Biological Data Relevant to the Evaluation of Carcinogenic Risk to Man (section 3)

As pointed out earlier in this introduction, the monographs are not intended to consider all reported studies. Although every effort was made to review the whole literature, some studies were purposely omitted (a) because of their inadequacy, as judged from previously described criteria[22-25] (e.g., too short a duration, too few animals, poor survival or too small a dose); (b) because they only confirmed findings which have already been fully described; or (c) because they were judged irrelevant for the purpose of the evaluation. However, in certain cases, reference is made to studies which did not meet established criteria of adequacy, particularly when this information was considered a useful supplement to other reports or when it may have been the only data available. This does not, however, imply acceptance of the adequacy of experimental designs in these cases.

In general, the data recorded in this section are summarized as given by the author; however, certain shortcomings of reporting or of experimental design are also mentioned, and minor comments by the Working Group are given in square brackets.

The essential comments by the Working Group are made in section 4, 'Comments on Data Reported and Evaluation'.

Carcinogenicity and related studies in animals: Mention is usually made of all routes of administration by which the compound has been tested and of all species in which relevant tests have been carried out. In most cases the animal strains are given; general characteristics of mouse strains have been reported in a recent review[26]. Quantitative data are given in so far as they will enable the reader to realize the order of magnitude of the effective doses. In general, the doses are indicated as they appear in the original paper; sometimes conversions have been made for better comparison.

Other relevant biological data: The reporting of metabolic data is restricted to studies showing the metabolic fate of the chemical in animals and man. Comparison of animal and human data is made when possible. Other metabolic information (e.g., absorption, storage and excretion) is given when the Working Group considered that it would enable the reader to have a better understanding of the fate of the compound in the body. When the carcinogenicity of known metabolites has been tested, this also is reported.

Some LD_{50}'s are given, and other data on toxicity are included, if considered relevant.

Mutagenicity data are also included, and the reasons for including such data and the principles adopted by the Working Group for selection of the data are outlined below.

Many, but not all, mutagens are carcinogens and *vice versa*; the exact level of correlation is still under investigation. Nevertheless, practical use may be made of the available mutagenicity test procedures that combine microbial, mammalian or other animal cell systems as genetic targets with an *in vitro* or *in vivo* metabolic activation system. The results of relatively rapid and inexpensive mutagenicity tests on non-human organisms may help to pre-screen chemicals and may also aid in the selection of the most relevant animal species in which to carry out long-term carcinogenicity tests on these chemicals.

In seeking to make predictive use of, and to provide an explanation for, the observed correlation between carcinogenicity and mutagenicity, the ultimate goal is to detect genetic changes in the complete range of cell types in humans; but this is not attainable at present.

The role of genetic alterations in chemical carcinogenesis is not known, and therefore consideration must be given to a variety of changes. Although nuclear DNA has been defined as the main cellular target for the induction of genetic changes, other relevant targets have been recognized, e.g., mitochondrial DNA, enzymes involved in DNA synthesis, repair and recombination, and the spindle apparatus. Tests to detect the genetic activity of chemicals, including gene mutation, structural and numerical chromosomal changes and mitotic recombination, are available for non-human models; but not all such tests can be applied at present to human cells.

There are many genetic indicators and metabolic activation systems available for detecting mutagenic activity; they all, however, have individual advantages and limitations. Ideally, an appropriate mutagenicity test system would include the full metabolic competency of the intact human.

Since the development or application of such a system appears to be impossible, the conclusion has been reached that a battery of test systems is needed in order to establish the mutagenic potential of chemicals.

Since many chemicals require metabolism to an active form, test systems which do not take this into account may fail to reveal the full range of genetic damage. Furthermore, since some reactive metabolites with a limited lifespan may fail to reach or to react with the genetic indicator, either because they are further metabolized to inactive compounds or because they react with other cellular constituents, mutagenicity tests in intact animals may give false negative results.

It is difficult in the present state of knowledge to select specific mutagenicity tests as being the most appropriate for the pre-screening of substances for possible carcinogenic activity. However, greater reliance may be placed on data obtained from those test systems which (a) permit the identification of the nature of induced genetic changes, and (b) demonstrate that the changes are transmitted to subsequent generations. Mutagenicity tests using organisms that are well-understood genetically, e.g., *Escherichia coli*, *Salmonella typhimurium*, *Saccharomyces* and *Drosophila*, meet these requirements.

Although a correlation has often been observed between the ability of a chemical to cause chromosome breakage and its ability to induce gene mutation, data on chromosomal breakage alone do not provide adequate evidence for mutagenicity, and therefore lesser weight should be given to pre-screening that is based on the use of peripheral leucocyte cultures.

Because of the complexity of factors that can contribute to reproductive failure, as well as the insensitivity of the method, the dominant lethal test in the mammal does not provide reliable data on mutagenicity.

A large-scale systematic screening of compounds to assess a correlation between mutagenicity and carcinogenicity has so far been carried out only with the bacterial/mammalian liver microsome system. Notwithstanding the demonstration of the mutagenicity of many known carcinogens to *Salmonella typhimurium* in the presence of liver microsomal systems, the possibility of false-negative and false-positive results must not be overlooked.

False negatives might arise as a consequence of mutagen specificity or from failure to achieve optimal conditions for activation *in vitro*. Alternative test systems must be used if there appear to be substantial reasons for suspecting that a chemical which is apparently non-mutagenic in a bacterial test system may nevertheless be potentially carcinogenic. Conversely, some chemicals found to be mutagenic in this test may not in fact have mutagenic activity in other systems.

For more detailed information, see references 27-34.

Observations in man: Case reports of cancer and epidemiological studies are summarized in this section.

Comments on Data Reported and Evaluation (section 4)

This section gives the critical view of the Working Group on the data reported. It should be read in conjunction with the 'General Remarks on the Substances Considered'.

Animal data: The animal species mentioned are those in which the carcinogenicity of the substances was clearly demonstrated, irrespective of the route of administration. In the case of inadequate studies, when mentioned, comments to that effect are included. The route of administration used in experimental animals that is similar to the possible human exposure (ingestion, inhalation and skin exposure) is given particular mention. In most cases tumour sites are also indicated. Experiments involving a possible action of the vehicle or a physical effect of the agent, such as in subcutaneous injection or bladder implantation studies, are also mentioned; however, the results of such tests require careful consideration, particularly if they are the only ones raising a suspicion of carcinogenicity. If the substance has produced tumours on pre-natal exposure or in single-dose experiments, this is also indicated. This sub-section should be read in the light of comments made in the section, 'Animal Data in Relation to the Evaluation of Risk to Man' of this introduction.

Human data: In some cases, a brief statement is made on the possible exposure of man. The significance of epidemiological studies and case reports is discussed, and the data are interpreted in terms of possible human risk.

References

1. IARC (1972) *IARC Monographs on the Evaluation of Carcinogenic Risk of Chemicals to Man, 1*, Lyon

2. IARC (1973) *IARC Monographs on the Evaluation of Carcinogenic Risk of Chemicals to Man, 2, Some Inorganic and Organometallic Compounds*, Lyon

3. IARC (1973) *IARC Monographs on the Evaluation of Carcinogenic Risk of Chemicals to Man, 3, Certain Polycyclic Aromatic Hydrocarbons and Heterocyclic Compounds*, Lyon

4. IARC (1974) *IARC Monographs on the Evaluation of Carcinogenic Risk of Chemicals to Man, 4, Some Aromatic Amines, Hydrazine and Related Substances, N-Nitroso Compounds and Miscellaneous Alkylating Agents*, Lyon

5. IARC (1974) *IARC Monographs on the Evaluation of Carcinogenic Risk of Chemicals to Man, 5, Some Organochlorine Pesticides*, Lyon

6. IARC (1974) *IARC Monographs on the Evaluation of Carcinogenic Risk of Chemicals to Man, 6, Sex Hormones*, Lyon

7. IARC (1974) *IARC Monographs on the Evaluation of Carcinogenic Risk of Chemicals to Man, 7, Some Anti-thyroid and Related Substances, Nitrofurans and Industrial Chemicals*, Lyon

8. IARC (1975) *IARC Monographs on the Evaluation of Carcinogenic Risk of Chemicals to Man, 8, Some Aromatic Azo Compounds*, Lyon

9. IARC (1975) *IARC Monographs on the Evaluation of Carcinogenic Risk of Chemicals to Man, 9, Some Aziridines, N-, S- and O-Mustards and Selenium*, Lyon

10. IARC (1976) *IARC Monographs on the Evaluation of Carcinogenic Risk of Chemicals to Man, 10, Some Naturally Occurring Substances*, Lyon

11. Hartwell, J.L. (1951) *Survey of compounds which have been tested for carcinogenic activity*, Washington DC, US Government Printing Office (Public Health Service Publication No. 149)

12. Shubik, P. & Hartwell, J.L. (1957) *Survey of compounds which have been tested for carcinogenic activity*, Washington DC, US Government Printing Office (Public Health Service Publication No. 149: Supplement 1)

13. Shubik, P. & Hartwell, J.L. (1969) *Survey of compounds which have been tested for carcinogenic activity*, Washington DC, US Government Printing Office (Public Health Service Publication No. 149: Supplement 2)

14. Carcinogenesis Program National Cancer Institute (1971) _Survey of compounds which have been tested for carcinogenic activity_ Washington DC, US Government Printing Office (Public Health Service Publication No. 149: 1968-1969)

15. Carcinogenesis Program National Cancer Institute (1973) _Survey of compounds which have been tested for carcinogenic activity,_ Washington DC, US Government Printing Office (Public Health Service Publication No. 149: 1961-1967)

16. Carcinogenesis Program National Cancer Institute (1974) _Survey of compounds which have been tested for carcinogenic activity,_ Washington DC, US Government Printing Office (Public Health Service Publication No. 149: 1970-1971)

17. WHO (1961) Fifth Report of the Joint FAO/WHO Expert Committee on Food Additives. Evaluation of carcinogenic hazard of food additives. _Wld Hlth Org. techn. Rep. Ser._, No. 220, pp. 5, 18, 19

18. WHO (1969) Report of a WHO Scientific Group. Principles for the testing and evaluation of drugs for carcinogenicity. _Wld Hlth Org. techn. Rep. Ser._, No. 426, pp. 19, 21, 22

19. WHO (1964) Report of a WHO Expert Committee. Prevention of cancer. _Wld Hlth Org. techn. Rep. Ser._, No. 276, pp. 29, 30

20. Stecher, P.G., ed. (1968) _The Merck Index_, 8th ed., Rahway, NJ, Merck & Co.

21. Weast, R.C., ed. (1975) _CRC Handbook of Chemistry and Physics,_ 56th ed., Cleveland, Ohio, Chemical Rubber Co.

22. WHO (1958) Second Report of the Joint FAO/WHO Expert Committee on Food Additives. Procedures for the testing of intentional food additives to establish their safety for use. _Wld Hlth Org. techn. Rep. Ser._, No. 144

23. WHO (1961) Fifth Report of the Joint FAO/WHO Expert Committee on Food Additives. Evaluation of carcinogenic hazard of food additives. _Wld Hlth Org. techn. Rep. Ser._, No. 220

24. WHO (1967) Scientific Group. Procedures for investigating intentional and unintentional food additives. _Wld Hlth Org. techn. Rep. Ser._, No. 348

25. UICC (1969) Carcinogenicity testing. _UICC techn. Rep. Ser._, _2_

26. Committee on Standardized Genetic Nomenclature for Mice (1972) Standardized nomenclature for inbred strains of mice. Fifth listing. _Cancer Res._, _32_, 1609-1646

27. Bartsch, H. & Grover, P.L. (1976) *Chemical carcinogenesis and mutagenesis*. In: Symington, T. & Carter, R.L., eds, *Scientific Foundations of Oncology*, Vol. IX, *Chemical Carcinogenesis*, London, Heinemann Medical Books Ltd, pp.334-342

28. Holländer, A., ed. (1971) *Chemical Mutagens: Principles and Methods for Their Detection*, Vols 1-3, New York, Plenum Press

29. Montesano, R. & Tomatis, L., eds (1974) Chemical Carcinogenesis Essays, *IARC Scientific Publications, No. 10*, Lyon, IARC

30. Ramel, C., ed. (1973) *Evaluation of genetic risks of environmental chemicals*, Report of a symposium held at Skokloster, Sweden, 1972, *Ambio Special Report No. 3*, Royal Swedish Academy of Sciences/Universitetsforlaget

31. Stoltz, D.R., Poirier, L.A., Irving, C.C., Stich, H.F., Weisburger, J.H. & Grice, H.C. (1974) Evaluation of short-term tests for carcinogenicity. *Toxicol. appl. Pharmacol., 29*, 157-180

32. WHO (1974) Report of a WHO Scientific Group. Assessment of the carcinogenicity and mutagenicity of chemicals. *Wld Hlth Org. techn. Rep. Ser., No. 546*

33. Montesano, R., Bartsch, H. & Tomatis, L., eds (1975) Screening Tests in Chemical Carcinogenesis, *IARC Scientific Publications, No. 12*, Lyon, IARC

34. Committee 17 (1975) Environmental mutagenic hazards. *Science, 187*, 503-514

GENERAL REMARKS ON THE SUBSTANCES CONSIDERED

New data concerning cadmium and nickel and their salts were considered, and the existing monographs (IARC, 1973) on these substances have been updated.

Most of the epoxides considered in this volume have commercial uses, and some are found in manufactured materials, food and air. Two epoxides which occur naturally, fusarenon-X and *cis*-9,10-epoxystearic acid, are also included. There is increasing documentation concerning the general chemical and biological reactivity of epoxides, although for some of them the carcinogenicity data are inadequate for evaluation. Epoxy resins and epoxidized vegetable oils are considered in these general remarks and not in specific monographs because they are of variable composition.

Other substances were selected for consideration because of their industrial importance and because they were suspected of being carcinogenic (i.e., benzyl chloride, β- and γ-butyrolactone, dinitrosopentamethylene-tetramine, 1,4-dioxane, ethylene sulphide, trichloroethylene and 4-vinyl-cyclohexene).

Volatile anaesthetics are considered because of two epidemiological surveys which indicate a cancer risk among people working in operating theatres; however, insufficient experimental data on the carcinogenicity of most of the anaesthetics (halogenated hydrocarbons or halogenated ethers) were available. Thus, the section 'General Considerations on Volatile Anaesthetics' includes a discussion of the cancer risk associated with these compounds. A separate monograph was prepared for trichloro-ethylene, since it is also widely used as an industrial solvent.

The Working Group also considered some other substances [bis(2-chloro-isopropyl)ether, butyl-*cis*-9,10-epoxystearate, 4-chloro-*ortho*-toluidine, chloroprene, nivalenol, styrene, tetrachloroethylene, *ortho*-toluidine and vinylidene chloride]. Monographs on these substances are not included in this volume, however, since the available animal and/or human data were insufficient for a proper consideration and since the Working Group was aware of animal and epidemiological studies in progress on some of these substances. In the light of such new data future Working Groups will reconsider these compounds. In this context the Working Group expressed concern over the long delay that sometimes occurs in the publication of important results.

Epoxides

Data on purity are lacking for some of these substances; some indication of possible contaminants can be obtained from methods of synthesis. Because of the low stability and high reactivity of certain of these compounds, knowledge of their fate in test media is essential for assessing their various biological effects.

No details of methods of analysis for certain specific epoxy compounds included in these monographs were available to the Working Group. Since most of these substances are volatile, however, gas chromatography can be employed for their determination. Colorimetric determinations by the measurement of periodate oxidation products (Mishmash & Meloan, 1972) and of reaction products with 4-(4'-nitrobenzyl)pyridine (Preussmann et al., 1969) are also applicable. Analytical methods for a number of epoxy compounds were given by Fishbein & Falk (1969).

The occurrence of epoxides in air has been reviewed (NAS-NRC, 1976); they can be formed metabolically by microsomal mono-oxygenases from aromatic or olefinic precursors (Daly et al., 1972; Oesch, 1973; Sims & Grover, 1974).

Hendry et al. (1951) and Van Duuren et al. (1967) discussed the relationship between carcinogenicity and chemical structure of these compounds.

Some epoxides react irreversibly with cellular macromolecules (Grover et al., 1971; Lawley & Jarman, 1972). Microsomal epoxide hydrase converts epoxides into dihydrodiols (Daly et al., 1972; Oesch, 1973; Sims & Grover, 1974); cytoplasmic glutathione S-epoxide transferases convert them into glutathione conjugates (Boyland & Chasseaud, 1969; Fjellstedt et al., 1973; Jerina et al., 1970a). Dihydrodiols are subsequently converted by cytoplasmic dihydrodiol dehydrogenase into catechols (Ayengar et al., 1959; Jerina et al., 1970b), which are further converted by catechol O-methyltransferases into guaiacols (Oesch, 1973). Both dihydrodiols and catechols are conjugated to form glucuronides and sulphates. The glutathione conjugates are converted by several steps into mercapturic acids (*N*-acetylcysteine conjugates) (Boyland *et al.*, 1961). Glucuronides, sulphates and mercapturic acids represent the major urinary and biliary metabolites of epoxides.

In addition to these enzymatic reactions, epoxides can undergo spontaneous rearrangements: arene oxides rearrange to phenols by the 'NIH-shift' (Daly *et al.*, 1972). Rearrangement of chlorinated alkene oxides was suggested to occur during the metabolism of trichloroethylene (Powell, 1945), and such rearrangements occur with several chlorinated ethylene oxides (Bonse *et al.*, 1975; Gross & Freiberg, 1969).

The relationship between chemical properties and biological effects of epoxides and other alkylating agents has been reviewed (Sawicki & Sawicki, 1969; Weil *et al.* 1963; Wheeler, 1962). Biological activity appears to be associated with their reaction with nucleophilic sites in cellular components, such as proteins and nucleic acids. Bifunctional alkylating agents (e.g., diepoxy compounds) may inactivate DNA templates by formation of interstrand cross-links which cause inhibition of DNA synthesis and toxic effects (Van Duuren & Goldschmidt, 1966). This type of interaction and their greater effect on rapidly dividing cells form the basis of the use of certain epoxy compounds as anti-cancer drugs.

Some epoxides have been shown to have radiomimetic activity; they also cause central nervous system depression (particularly of the respiratory centre), irritation of skin and mucous membranes and skin sensitization.

Due to their alkylating properties, many epoxides have shown mutagenic activity in a number of biological systems. The majority of these studies have been performed with bacteria. Most of the changes to DNA caused by these compounds produce base-pair substitutions which give rise to genetically transmissible alterations.

Epoxy resins and epoxidized vegetable oils

Only chemically well-defined epoxy compounds are considered in these monographs, but any account of the carcinogenic risk of epoxides to man would be incomplete without consideration of two classes of epoxide-containing materials, namely, epoxidized vegetable oils and epoxy resins. These materials are produced in large quantities, so that people can be exposed during both their manufacture and use.

Epoxy resins

Of the many different materials used to produce epoxy resins, those made from epichlorohydrin and bisphenol-A (diphenylol propane) accounted for approximately 90% of the 113 million kg of all unmodified epoxy resins produced in the US in 1974 (The Society of the Plastics Industry, Inc., 1975). In commercial applications these resins are converted to cured resins (using catalysts or reactive hardeners) by cross-linking reactions which convert essentially all of the epoxy groups to other structures and yield resins with the desired physical properties. About half of the amount produced in the US in 1974 was used in protective coatings. They are also used for fibre-reinforced laminates, floor coverings and adhesives, some of which are sold for use by the public.

An uncured epoxy resin (average molecular weight, 300), derived from an aliphatic diol and epichlorhydrin, was tested in male C3H mice by skin painting on the clipped nape of the neck with a 5% solution in acetone. Of 13 mice given thrice weekly applications, 4 developed squamous-cell carcinomas of the skin; in 20 mice given once weekly skin paintings, 1 sarcoma at the site of application was seen. This product also produced local sarcomas in 9/23 male Long-Evans rats given 3 s.c. injections of a 10% solution in propylene glycol at weekly intervals. Another epoxy resin, based on bisphenol-A and epichlorohydrin (average molecular weight, 350), did not produce skin tumours in male C3H mice when applied thrice weekly as a 5% solution in acetone. In male Long-Evans rats, local sarcomas occurred in 4/16 animals given 3 s.c. injections of the resin as a 50% solution in propylene glycol at weekly intervals. The animals in all experiments were observed for 2 years. No tumours occurred in 30 vehicle-treated control mice and rats (Hine *et al.*, 1958).

Epoxidized vegetable oils

Epoxidized soya bean oil, the most important of the commercially epoxidized vegetable oils [US production was 46.5 million kg in 1974 (US

International Trade Commission, 1975)], is used at levels of 1.5-3% in resin for many polyvinyl chloride (PVC) formulations as a heat and light stabilizer. It is used at higher concentrations as a plasticizer in PVC formulations occurring in such products as automobiles, furniture, floor coverings, packaging film and coatings for wire.

Experiments involving chronic feeding of epoxidized soya bean oil to C57 black mice have been reported (Kotin & Falk, 1963) but were inadequate for evaluation. *cis*-9,10-Epoxystearic acid, a constituent of epoxidized linseed oil, is considered in a separate monograph.

5. References

Ayengar, P.K., Hayaischi, O., Nakajima, M. & Tomida, I. (1959) Enzymatic aromatization of 3,5-cyclohexadiene-1,2-diol. Biochim. biophys. acta, 33, 111-119

Bonse, G., Urban, T., Reichert, D. & Henschler, D. (1975) Chemical reactivity, metabolic oxirane formation and biological reactivity of chlorinated ethylenes in the isolated perfused rat liver preparation. Biochem. Pharmacol., 24, 1829-1834

Boyland, E. & Chasseaud, L.F. (1969) The role of glutathione and glutathione S-transferases in mercapturic acid biosynthesis. Advanc. Enzymol., 32, 173-219

Boyland, E., Ramsay, G.S. & Sims, P. (1961) The secretion of metabolites of naphthalene, 1:2-dihydronaphthalene and 1:2-epoxy-1:2:3:4-tetrahydronaphthalene in rat bile. Biochem. J., 78, 376-384

Daly, J.W., Jerina, D.M. & Witkop, B. (1972) Arene oxides and the NIH shift: the metabolism, toxicity and carcinogenicity of aromatic compounds. Experientia, 28, 1129-1149

Fishbein, L. & Falk, H. (1969) Chromatography of alkylating agents. II. Nitrosamines, epoxides, lactones, methane sulfonates and miscellaneous derivatives. Chromat. Rev., 11, 365-445

Fjellstedt, T.A., Allen, R.H., Duncan, B.K. & Jacoby, W.B. (1973) Enzymatic conjugation of epoxides with glutathione. J. biol. Chem., 248, 3702-3707

Gross, H. & Freiberg, J. (1969) Zur Existenz von Chloroäthylenoxid. J. prakt. Chem., 311, 506-510

Grover, P.L., Forrester, J.A. & Sims, P. (1971) Reactivity of the K-region epoxides of some polycyclic hydrocarbons towards the nucleic acids and proteins of BHK 21 cells. Biochem. Pharmacol., 20, 1297-1302

Hendry, J.A., Homer, R.F., Rose, F.L. & Walpole, A.L. (1951) Cytotoxic agents. II. Bis-epoxides and related compounds. Brit. J. Pharmacol., 6, 235-255

Hine, C.H., Guzman, R.J., Coursey, M.M., Wellington, J.S. & Anderson, H.H. (1958) An investigation of the oncogenic activity of two representative epoxy resins. Cancer Res., 18, 20-26

IARC (1973) IARC Monographs on the Evaluation of Carcinogenic Risk of Chemicals to Man, 2, Some inorganic and organometallic compounds, Lyon, pp.74-99, 126-149

Jerina, D.M., Daly, J.W., Witkop, B., Zaltzman-Nirenberg, P. & Udenfriend, S. (1970a) 1,2-Naphthalene oxide as an intermediate in the microsomal hydroxylation of naphthalene. Biochemistry, 9, 147-155

Jerina, D.M., Ziffer, H. & Daly, J.W. (1970b) The role of the arene oxide-oxepin system in the metabolism of aromatic substrates. IV. Stereochemical considerations of dihydrodiol formation and dehydrogenation. J. Amer. chem. Soc., 92, 1056-1061

Kotin, P. & Falk, H.L. (1963) Organic peroxides, hydrogen peroxide, epoxides and neoplasia. Rad. Res. Suppl., 3, 193-211

Lawley, P.D. & Jarman, M. (1972) Alkylation by propylene oxide of deoxyribonucleic acid, adenine, guanosine and deoxyguanylic acid. Biochem. J., 126, 893-900

Mishmash, H.E. & Meloan, C.E. (1972) Indirect spectrophotometric determination of nanomole quantities of oxiranes. Analyt. Chem., 44, 835-836

NAS-NRC (National Academy of Sciences-National Research Council) (1976) Vapor Phase Organic Air Pollutants, Washington DC, US Government Printing Office (in press)

Oesch, F. (1973) Mammalian epoxide hydrases. Inducible enzymes catalysing the inactivation of carcinogenic and cytotoxic metabolites derived from aromatic and olefinic compounds. Xenobiotica, 3, 305-340

Powell, J.F. (1945) Trichloroethylene: absorption, elimination and metabolism. Brit. J. industr. Med., 2, 142-145

Preussmann, R., Schneider, H. & Epple, F. (1969) Untersuchungen zum Nachweis alkylierender Agentien. II. Der Nachweis verschiedener Klassen alkylierender Agentien mit einer Modifikation der Farbreaktion mit 4-(4'-Nitrobenzyl)-pyridin (NBP). Arzneimittelforsch., 19, 1059-1073

Sawicki, E. & Sawicki, C.R. (1969) Analysis of alkylating agents: applications to air pollution. Ann. N.Y. Acad. Sci., 163, 895-920

Sims, P. & Grover, P.L. (1974) Epoxides in polycyclic aromatic hydrocarbon metabolism and carcinogenesis. Advanc. Cancer Res., 20, 165-294

The Society of the Plastics Industry, Inc. (1975) 1974 Final Monthly Statistical Report, Plastic and Resin Materials, SPI Committee on Resin Statistics, March 21, New York, Ernst & Ernst, p. 3

US International Trade Commission (1975) Preliminary Report on US Production of Selected Synthetic Organic Chemicals, Preliminary Totals, 1974, S.O.C. Series C/P-75-1, Washington DC, US Government Printing Office, p.2

Van Duuren, B.L. & Goldschmidt, B.M. (1966) Carcinogenicity of epoxides, lactones and peroxy compounds. III. Biological activity and chemical reactivity. J. med. Chem., 9, 77-79

Van Duuren, B.L., Langseth, L., Goldschmidt, B.M. & Orris, L. (1967) Carcinogenicity of epoxides, lactones and peroxy compounds. VI. Structure and carcinogenic activity. J. nat. Cancer Inst., 39, 1217-1228

Weil, C.S., Condra, N., Haun, C. & Striegel, J.A. (1963) Experimental carcinogenicity and acute toxicity of representative epoxides. *Amer. industr. Hyg. Ass. J.*, 24, 305-315

Wheeler, G.P. (1962) Studies related to the mechanisms of action of cytotoxic alkylating agents: a review. *Cancer Res.*, 22, 651-688

THE MONOGRAPHS

CADMIUM AND CADMIUM COMPOUNDS*

Cadmium and cadmium compounds were first considered by an IARC Working Group in 1972 (IARC, 1973). Since that time new data have become available, and these are included in the present monograph and have been taken into consideration in the evaluation.

A general review of cadmium and its compounds has been published (Fulkerson et al., 1973), and a WHO Environmental Health Criteria Document is in preparation.

1. Chemical and Physical Data

1.1 Synonyms, trade names and formulae

Table I

(Chemical Abstracts names are underlined.)

Chemical Name	Chem. Abstr. Reg. Serial No.	Synonyms	Formula
Cadmium	7440-43-9	C.I. No. 77180	Cd
Cadmium acetate	543-90-8	Acetic acid, cadmium salt; C.I. No. 77185	$Cd(CH_3COO)_2$
Cadmium carbonate	513-78-0	Carbonic acid, cadmium salt (1:1); cadmium monocarbonate; otavite; Chemcarb	$CdCO_3$
Cadmium chloride	10108-64-2	Cadmium dichloride	$CdCl_2$
Cadmium fluoborate	14486-19-2	Borate, (1-)tetrafluoro-, cadmium salt (2:1)	$Cd(BF_4)_2$
Cadmium fluoride	7790-79-6		CdF_2

---

*Considered by the Working Group, December 1975

Cadmium molybdate	13972-68-4	Molybdic acid, cadmium salt (1:1)	$CdMoO_4$
Cadmium nitrate	10325-94-7	Nitric acid, cadmium (2+) salt (1:2)	$Cd(NO_3)_2$
Cadmium oxide	1306-19-0		CdO
Cadmium sulphate	10124-36-4	Sulphuric acid, cadmium salt (1:1)	$CdSO_4$
Cadmium sulphide	1306-23-6	Aurora yellow; cadmopur golden yellow N; cadmopur yellow; C.I. No. 77199; C.I. pigment orange 20; C.I. pigment yellow 37; greenockite Capsebon	CdS

1.2 Chemical and physical properties

Physical properties of the cadmium compounds considered in this monograph are given, when available, in Table II. Additional information on solubility is given below.

Cadmium metal - soluble in dilute nitric acid and in sulphuric acid

Cadmium acetate - very soluble in water and soluble in methanol

Cadmium carbonate - insoluble in water (Schindler, 1967), soluble in acids, ammonium salts and potassium cyanide

Cadmium chloride - soluble in water (140 g/100 ml at 20°C; 150 g/100 ml at 100°C) and slightly soluble in methanol (1.7 g/100 ml at 15.5°C) and ethanol (1.5 g/100 ml at 15°C); it forms hydrates containing 1, 2.5 and 4 molecules of water, respectively.

Cadmium fluoborate - extremely hygroscopic and very soluble in water and 95% ethanol (Stacey *et al.*, 1960)

Cadmium fluoride - soluble in hydrogen fluoride (0.2 g/100 g at 14.2°C) (Jache & Cady, 1952) and in water (3.5 g/100 ml at 25°C) (Pascal, 1959)

Cadmium molybdate - slightly soluble in water and soluble in acids, ammonium hydroxide and potassium cyanide

Table II [a]

Chemical Name	Atomic/mol. weight	Melting-point °C	Boiling-point °C	Crystal system	Density g/cm³	Refractive index n_D^{20}
Cadmium	112.40	320.9	765	hexagonal, silver-white metal	8.642^{20}	1.8 at 578 nm [c]
Cadmium acetate	230.50	256			2.341	
Cadmium carbonate	172.41			trigonal, white powder	4.258^4	
Cadmium chloride	183.32	568		hexagonal, colourless	4.047^{25}	1.65 at 589.3 nm
Cadmium fluoride	150.40		1758	cubic, white	6.33 [b]	1.56 at 589.3 nm
Cadmium molybdate	272.34			yellow plates	5.347	
Cadmium nitrate	236.41	350		colourless solid	2.45 [d]	
Cadmium oxide	128.40	900 (dec.)	1559 (subl.)	cubic, brown	8.15	2.49 at 670.8 nm
Cadmium sulphate	208.46	1000		rhombic, white	4.691_4^{20}	
Cadmium sulphide	144.46	1750 at 100 atm	980 (subl. in N₂)	hexagonal, yellow-orange	4.82	2.506; 2.529 at 589.3 nm

[a] Data from Weast (1975) unless otherwise specified
[b] From Haendler & Bernard (1951)
[c] From Lyman (1961)
[d] From Pascal (1959)

Cadmium nitrate - very soluble in water (109 g/100 ml at $0°C$; 326 g/100 ml at $60°C$; 682 g/100 ml at $100°C$) (Weast, 1975)

Cadmium oxide - insoluble in water and alkalis but soluble in acids and solutions of ammonium salts (Greene, 1974)

Cadmium sulphate - soluble in water (75.5 g/100 ml at $0°C$; 60.8 g/100 ml at $100°C$) (Weast, 1975) but barely soluble in methanol and ethanol (Pascal, 195

Cadmium sulphide - soluble in acids and in ammonium hydroxide (Greene, 1974) but barely soluble in water (0.00013 g/100 ml at $18°C$) (Weast, 1975)

1.3 Technical products and impurities

Tentative specifications for cadmium metal issued in 1966 by the American Society for Testing and Materials (US Bureau of Mines, 1970) made the following requirements:

Element	Percentage
Cadmium (by difference), minimum	99.90
Zinc, maximum	.035
Copper, maximum	.015
Lead, maximum	.025
Tin, maximum	.01
Silver, maximum	.01
Antimony, maximum	.001
Arsenic, maximum	.003
Thallium, maximum	.003

Cadmium sponge when dispatched to customers has a moisture content of about 25% when packaged in bags and 35% when packaged in drums. Even with this precaution, substantial oxidation occurs, and typical cadmium contents on a dry basis are 86% in bags and 92% in drums. A pure form of cadmium for electronic uses contains 0.001% or less of impurities.

Cadmium acetate is usually available as the hydrate $Cd(CH_3COO)_2 \cdot 2H_2O$ in technical or reagent grades.

Cadmium carbonate is available in a commercial grade which has a purity of about 98%, lead, zinc and iron being present as impurities. Higher purity grades are available for special applications.

Commercial cadmium chloride is a mixture of hydrates that approximates to the dihydrate ($CdCl_2 \cdot 2H_2O$). The commercial grade of cadmium chloride available in the US typically contains about 51% cadmium and 0.005% each of iron and copper. There are higher purity grades available for specialized applications such as photographic chemicals and phosphors.

Cadmium nitrate with a purity greater than 99% can be obtained; typical impurities are chloride (0.005%), sulphate (0.005%), copper (0.005%), iron (0.002%), lead (0.005%), zinc (0.05%) and arsenic (0.001%).

The commercial grade of cadmium oxide available in the US has a reported purity of 99.7%, with lead and thallium as detectable impurities.

Commercial grade cadmium sulphate reportedly contains about 49.5% cadmium; the theoretical cadmium content of $CdSO_4$ is 53.5%.

Because cadmium sulphide and cadmium sulphide-containing materials are used principally for their physical properties rather than for their chemical ones, the usual measures of product grading are seldom used. Although the commercial grade of cadmium sulphide, when not otherwise specified as a pigment or a phosphor, typically contains 98.8% cadmium sulphide and 0.7% cadmium sulphate, most products in which it occurs are more complex. Thus, cadmium yellow pigments are cadmium sulphide-zinc sulphide mixtures; cadmium lithopone pigments are co-precipitates of cadmium sulphide and barium sulphate; cadmium sulphoselenides are varied mixtures of cadmium sulphide, cadmium selenide and selenium sulphide; and the so-called mercadium pigments contain mercuric sulphide in combination with cadmium sulphide. The cadmium sulphide used in phosphors is usually a mixture with zinc sulphide and contains trace amounts of activators such as silver, copper or nickel.

2. Production, Use, Occurrence and Analysis

For important background information on this section, see preamble, p. 19.

2.1 Production and use

Cadmium: The principal sources of cadmium are the sintering of flue dusts and the roasting of zinc ores. Some cadmium metal is also recovered as a by-product of the purification by distillation of slag zinc.

World production of cadmium was about 16.5 million kg in 1970 and had increased to 17 million kg by 1973 (Hague, 1973; Teworte, 1973, 1975). US production in 1973 was 3360 thousand kg (Hague, 1973).

Canada, Japan, US, USSR and Zaire accounted for 74% of the world production in 1965. Other countries with appreciable production include Australia, Austria, Belgium, Bulgaria, Federal Republic of Germany, France, German Democratic Republic, Honduras, Ireland, Italy, Mexico, The Netherlands, Norway, Peru, Poland, Spain, Sweden, Yugoslavia and Zambia (Fairbridge, 1974; US Bureau of Mines, 1975).

In 1973, US imports of cadmium metal were 1.76 million kg and of cadmium ore and flue dust, 793 thousand kg. In the same year, US exports were 139 thousand kg (US Bureau of Mines, 1975).

Demand for cadmium in the US has averaged 5.67 million kg over the last few years and has been used in the following ways: 49% in metal plating, 18% in plastics stabilizers, 14% in pigments and 19% in miscellaneous uses (nickel-cadmium batteries, alloys) (Bureau of National Affairs, Inc., 1975).

Nearly all cadmium electroplating is carried out in baths formulated from cadmium metal and cadmium oxide dissolved in a sodium cyanide solution, using a cadmium anode. The baths provide about 20% of the total amount of cadmium used in electroplating; the metal anodes account for the remaining 80%. The most important applications of this electroplating are in automotive and aircraft parts, electronic parts, marine equipment and industrial machinery. Cadmium electroplate, primarily on steel, is superior to that of zinc in providing resistance to corrosion. A general review of cadmium electroplating is given by Walker (1974).

The next largest use for cadmium is in the production of cadmium compounds that serve as stabilizers for plastics. The most common stabilizers are mixtures of cadmium and barium salts of long-chain fatty acids.

Another use of cadmium is in the preparation of cadmium sulphides, cadmium selenides and mixtures containing these salts for use as pigments (including phosphors). The phosphors require very pure starting materials, and cadmium oxide is preferred as the cadmium source.

Cadmium is used as the negative electrode in nickel-cadmium storage batteries found in industrial equipment, motor vehicles and many rechargeable household and biomedical appliances.

Cadmium-containing alloys are used for bearings where the high speeds and temperatures are excessive for tin or lead alloys. Such bearing alloys contain about 99% cadmium in combinations with nickel, silver and/or copper. Cadmium alloys used for soldering aluminium contain 10-95% cadmium, with zinc or silver as the other elements. Low-melting alloys of cadmium contain 8-40% of this metal in combination with bismuth, indium, tin and/or lead, and these alloys are used in a variety of applications (e.g., fire-protection fusible links, fusible cores for foundry moulds, holding irregular parts for machining, bending pipes and thin sections, soldering and sealing).

Other uses of cadmium that consume minor quantities include alloys for neutron shields and control rods for nuclear reactors. Spongy cadmium is used in the laboratory for the determination of nitrate.

Cadmium acetate: This compound can be prepared by treating cadmium nitrate with acetic anhydride (Stecher, 1968).

It is used to produce iridescent effects on porcelains and pottery and as a reagent for determination of sulphur, selenium and tellurium in cadmium electroplating (Stecher, 1968). It is also used in dyeing and printing textiles and in the purification of mercaptans from crude oils and gasolines (Greene, 1974).

Cadmium carbonate: Cadmium carbonate can be prepared by absorption of carbon dioxide in cadmium hydroxide solution, and this is believed to be the main commercial process.

Its major use is believed to be in fungicides. Cadmium carbonate is applied as a lawn and turf fungicide in concentrations of 3.0 and 5.3% as a wettable powder in combination with organic fungicides. The next most significant use is in the preparation of high-purity, specialized chemicals such as phosphors.

Cadmium chloride: The chloride is made by dissolving cadmium metal in hydrochloric acid and evaporating to dryness in a stream of hydrogen chloride gas or by dissolving cadmium oxide or carbonate in hydrochloric acid.

It is believed that pesticides are the largest single use of the commercial grade and that higher purity cadmium chloride is used increasingly in photographic materials and phosphors. It is used in non-pasture turf fungicides.

Minor uses for the chloride include its applications in dyeing and in calico-printing of textiles, in the manufacture of thermoionic emission coatings for electronic vacuum tubes, as a lubricant ingredient and in the manufacture of special mirrors.

Cadmium fluoborate: This compound is prepared from aqueous solutions of fluoboric acid and cadmium metal, carbonate or oxide; it is the hexahydrate form (Stacey *et al.*, 1960). Conventional methods of dehydration result in partial hydrolysis of the fluoborate ion and loss of volatile acidic components. It is more convenient and economical to supply 40-50% aqueous solutions (Halbedel, 1966).

Solutions of cadmium fluoborate are used in electroplating of metals.

Cadmium fluoride: Cadmium fluoride can be prepared by the reaction of cadmium carbonate with hydrofluoric acid. Its characteristics are similar to those of zinc fluoride, for which it may be substituted in certain phosphors. It is used as a glass ingredient and in nuclear reactor controls.

Cadmium molybdate: The molybdate forms when a solution of cadmium nitrate is treated with an alkaline molybdate solution (Sneed & Brasted, 1955). No information was available concerning its commercial uses.

Cadmium nitrate: Cadmium nitrate can be prepared by reacting cadmium oxide with nitric acid. It forms both a dihydrate and a tetrahydrate. The tetrahydrate, which is the major commercial form, is used principally in the manufacture of nickel-cadmium batteries. It has also been used as a turf fungicide.

Cadmium oxide: This compound is made commercially by distilling cadmium metal from a graphite retort and allowing the vapour to react with air.

Electroplating appears to be the largest use for cadmium oxide. Other important applications are in the manufacture of cadmium electrodes for alkaline storage batteries and in the synthesis of other cadmium salts.

Cadmium sulphate: The sulphate is made commercially as both the anhydrous ($CdSO_4$) and the hydrated salt ($3CdSO_4.8H_2O$). The usual commercial production of these materials involves dissolution of the metal, oxide, carbonate or sulphide in sulphuric acid with subsequent cooling or evaporation to precipitate the salt. Cadmium sulphate is also made as an intermediate in the recovery of cadmium from zinc ore.

The principal uses of cadmium sulphate are in the manufacture of cadmium salts of long-chain fatty acids used as stabilizers for plastics (especially polyvinyl chloride) and in the manufacture of cadmium sulphide pigments (including phosphors), of cadmium lithopone pigments and of cadmium sulphoselenide pigments. Its use in medicinal preparations has been discontinued owing to its toxicity.

Cadmium sulphide: Cadmium sulphide is produced commercially by the reaction of hydrogen sulphide gas with a cadmium salt (usually cadmium sulphate).

Almost all of the cadmium sulphide produced in the US is used in pigments (including phosphors). These pigments, which range in colour from yellow to deep maroon, are used principally when heat stability (e.g., in plastics, coloured vulcanized rubber and some epoxy resins), alkali resistance (printing inks) and resistance to hydrogen sulphide blackening (paints and artists' colours) are needed. Other materials for which cadmium sulphide pigments have been found useful include glass, ceramics, textiles and paper.

The principal phosphor use of cadmium sulphide is in cathode-ray tube screens. Minor quantities are used in a variety of applications that benefit from the low energy levels required to obtain visible light from this chemical. Phosphorescent tapes and markers, watch and instrument dials, interior decorations and theatrical effects are common uses. It is also used in X-ray fluorescent screens and body temperature gradient detectors.

Cadmium sulphide has been used as the active ingredient of shampoos designed for use in the treatment of seborrhoeic dermatitis of the scalp.

2.2 Occurrence

Reviews of the occurrence of cadmium in the environment have been published (Friberg *et al.*, 1974, 1975; Organization for Economic Cooperation and Development, 1975).

<u>Natural environment</u>: Cadmium is a relatively rare element in the earth's crust. Greenockite (cadmium sulphide) is the most common of its minerals, and it can be found in weathered ores as otavite (cadmium carbonate). In both forms it is associated with zinc and lead-zinc ores and is recovered as a by-product in their refining. Other minerals that contain cadmium are hawleyite, CdS; xanthocroite, $CdS(H_2O)_x$; cadmoselite, CdSe; and monteporrite, CdO (Fairbridge, 1974). Trace quantities of cadmium are also found in coals and oils.

<u>Air</u>: Cadmium can enter the air from a variety of manufacturing operations that involve either cadmium itself (e.g., production of copper-cadmium alloys) or zinc that contains cadmium as an impurity (e.g., smelting operations, galvanizing of steel). Cadmium can also enter the atmosphere when cadmium-plated scrap steel is remelted or from the incineration of waste plastics containing cadmium stabilizers and pigments. Smelting operations reportedly account for 87% of emissions to air, remelting of cadmium-plated steel for 9% and incineration for only 4% (Bureau of National Affairs, Inc., 1975).

Cadmium oxide and cadmium sulphate can also be found in atmospheric emissions from thermal processes involving cadmium.

In rural areas cadmium concentrations in ambient air are generally below 3 ng/m^3, but in large cities the yearly average may be up to 50 ng/m^3. In the vicinity of cadmium-emitting industries weekly or monthly means of about 500 ng/m^3 have been recorded (Friberg *et al.*, 1974).

<u>Cigarette smoke</u>: Determinations of cadmium in cigarette tobacco indicate a level of 1.7 µg per cigarette. As much as 10% of the cadmium may pass into the mainstream smoke (Szadkowski *et al.*, 1969). For a heavy

smoker this could add significantly to the daily cadmium intake: it is estimated that smokers who inhale 20 cigarettes per day accumulate 0.5 mg cadmium in one year (i.e., about 1.5 µg/day) (Lewis et al., 1972).

Occupational exposure: Exposure to cadmium has been high in the past: cadmium concentrations of several milligrams per m^3 of air were reported (Friberg, 1950; Petrovic & Kalember, 1969; Petrovic et al., 1968; Tarasenko & Vorobjeva, 1972). In recent years, possible improvements to the working environment have been proposed in order to reduce exposure, and Piscator et al. (1976) reported that in the accumulator factory studied by Friberg (1950) present air concentrations of cadmium are about 0.04 mg/m^3.

The concentration of cadmium oxide in the pre-mould department of a smelter ranged from 0.074-0.09 mg/m^3, and 1.1 mg/m^3 were found in the retort department (Lemen et al., 1976). Cadmium sulphide has also been found as a contaminant in working atmospheres, at concentrations generally less than 0.1 mg/m^3 (Harada, 1973). Concentrations of 0.08-25 mg/m^3 cadmium sulphate have been reported in the USSR (Tarasenko & Vorobjeva, 1972).

Water: Cadmium can enter surface waters from natural sources and from a variety of manufacturing operations that involve either cadmium itself (e.g., electroplating for corrosion protection) or zinc that contains a cadmium impurity (e.g., galvanizing of steel). It can enter the aqueous environment when spent solutions from plating operations are discarded. Ore tailings and washings from the production of refined cadmium metal are also potential sources of cadmium in nearby surface waters. Another source is the application of phosphate fertilizers, which have been found to contains traces of cadmium.

The level in non-polluted city water is less than 1 µg/l, but, as a result of industrial discharge and of the use of metal or plastic pipes, this level may increase to 10 µg/l (Friberg et al., 1974). It has been reported (Yamagata & Shigematsu, 1970) that in polluted rivers cadmium is often undetectable in the water itself but that high concentrations can be found in bottom sediments. Cadmium salts, such as cadmium carbonate, cadmium chloride and cadmium sulphate, may appear in surface waters as a result of run-off from industrial processes.

Soil and uptake in plants: In non-polluted areas, cadmium concentrations in soil are generally below 1 µg/g; whereas in polluted areas in Japan, concentrations of 1-70 µg have been found in rice fields (Friberg *et al.*, 1974). Both superphosphate fertilizers and sewage sludge used as fertilizer may add considerable quantities of cadmium to soil. Two important foodstuffs, wheat and rice, have been shown to have increased uptakes of cadmium when grown in soil containing large amounts (Friberg *et al.*, 1974).

Sources of soil pollution by cadmium have been estimated as follows: remelt steel operations (25%), stabilizers (24%), pigments (18%), batteries (6%), alloys and miscellaneous uses (12%), sewer sludge landfill (8%), sewer sludge incineration (3%) and solid waste incineration (4%) (Bureau of National Affairs, Inc., 1975).

Air, water, soil: The relative significance of some of the above applications in the US in 1968 has been estimated (Fulkerson *et al.*, 1973; US Environmental Protection Agency, 1975), and the results are given in Table III.

In principle, all of the cadmium and/or its salts, such as cadmium chloride, used as stabilizers and pigments in plastics could enter the environment, a process particularly facilitated by incineration. Thus, disposal of plastics could contribute to pollution by cadmium.

Food: There is little doubt that food is the main source of cadmium intake in non-occupationally exposed persons. The presence of cadmium in a wide range of both fresh and tinned foodstuffs has been reported by Klein & Wichmann (1945) and by Friberg *et al.* (1974, 1975). Schroeder & Balassa (1961) suggested that the main intake in the US diet was from sea-foods and grain products; vegetables were another source (Schroeder & Balassa, 1963).

Meat, eggs, fish and milk products generally have a low content of cadmium, less than 0.01 µg/g wet weight, whereas internal organs, especially liver and kidney, may contain much more; concentrations of up to 1 µg/g wet

Table III

Source	Quantity processed (thousand kg of cadmium)	Emissions to	Estimated emissions (thousand kg)
Primary processing			
Ore extraction	2150	Air Water, soil	0.2 Not available
Ore concentration and metal production	5800	Air	950
Conversion of metal to products	6000	Air	15
Product use	Not available	Air, water, soil	16
Recycle or disposal	–	Air, water, soil	1000
Miscellaneous			
Fossil fuel combustion	310	Air	90–320
Phosphate fertilizer application	20	Water, soil	Up to 22
Motor oil use	–	Air, water, soil	0.8

weight have been reported in animal organs. Some salmon meat was reported to contain more than 3 µg/g cadmium (Friberg et al., 1974), however, the analytical method used was not reported; internal organs from fish and shellfish may also contain high amounts (Banat et al., 1972; Oelschlaeger & Bestenlehner, 1975).

Vegetable products generally contain more cadmium than do animal products. Rice and wheat, two important foodstuffs, may contain from 0.01-01 µg/g in areas regarded as non-polluted; but in polluted areas in Japan, cadmium concentrations of 0.1-1 µg/g have commonly been found (Friberg et al., 1974).

The following table gives a comparison of the daily intakes in several countries (Friberg et al., 1974):

Country	µg Cd/day
Czechoslovakia	60
Federal Republic of Germany	48
Japan (non-polluted area)	47-59
Romania	38-64
US	4-92

General human exposure: In the general population, the main exposure is *via* food; and, except in the vicinity of some cadmium-emitting industries, cadmium in the ambient air does not contribute significantly. The daily intake *via* drinking-water is generally low but may be higher in contaminated areas or when cadmium-containing material contaminates tap-water. Smoking involves the inhalation of relatively small amounts of cadmium; but since it is highly absorbed from the lungs, in heavy smokers the absorbed amount may be of the same magnitude as that absorbed from food.

2.3 Analysis

General reviews of the analytical methods for cadmium are given by Friberg et al. (1974, 1975). An evaluation of analytical techniques for trace metals, including cadmium, in marine waters has been published (Lai, 1974).

The most common method is atomic absorption spectrophotometry, both flame and flameless methods. Extraction into organic solvents, ion-exchange separation or other methods of pre-treatment are often necessary. Blood, urine and some foodstuffs, in which cadmium concentrations are normally extremely low, previously presented analytical problems; interference from salts, e.g., sodium chloride, was the major problem; and many of the earlier data on the occurrence of cadmium in different media cannot be relied upon. During the last few years many of these analytical difficulties seem to have been overcome, and it is now possible to determine by flameless methods concentrations of less than 1 ng/g in blood and urine and less than 10 ng/g in foods (Kjellström et al., 1974a,b; Linnman et al., 1973).

Other useful techniques are neutron activation (Linnman et al., 1973; Ljunggren et al., 1971) and emission spectroscopy (Tipton et al., 1963). Anodic stripping voltametry and other electrochemical methods appear to be very useful for determination of cadmium in water (Whitnack & Sasselli, 1969), but more data are needed to evaluate their usefulness for the determination of cadmium in biological samples. The dithizone method (Church, 1947), which was previously the most commonly used method, is accurate, but the sensitivity is relatively low.

3. Biological Data Relevant to the Evaluation of Carcinogenic Risk to Man

Recent reviews on the biological action of cadmium are those of Flick et al. (1971), Friberg et al. (1974, 1975) and WHO (1972). Three general reviews on metal carcinogenesis which include cadmium are available (Furst & Haro, 1969; Sunderman, 1971, 1976).

3.1 Carcinogenicity and related studies in animals

(a) *Oral administration*

Mouse: Schroeder et al. (1964) observed no more tumours in 48 male and 39 female Swiss mice given cadmium acetate as 5 µg/ml Cd in their drinking-water for life than in 44 male and 60 female controls. The mean survival times were 814 days in the treated groups and 957 days in the control group in males and 904 and 966 days in females, respectively [The Working Group noted that the experimental dose level used was too low for carcinogenic evaluation. It was also noted that the concentrations in liver and kidney were below those generally seen in adult human beings].

Levy et al. (1975) gave 3 groups, each consisting of 50 male Swiss mice, weekly doses of cadmium sulphate by stomach tube (0.44, 0.88 and 1.75 mg/kg bw Cd) for 18 months, at which time the experiment was terminated. A control group of 150 mice was used. There were no differences between exposed animals and controls with regard to general health or tumour incidence. Special attention was paid to the prostate, but neoplastic lesions were not seen in that organ. Cadmium concentrations in organs were not reported.

Rat: Kanisawa & Schroeder (1969a) gave 47 Long-Evans rats cadmium acetate as 5 µg/ml Cd in the drinking-water for life. The tumour incidence was comparable with that in 34 controls. Schroeder et al. (1965) also found similar tumour incidences in 50 male and 46 female Long-Evans rats given cadmium acetate as 5 µg/ml Cd in their drinking-water for life and in 42 male and 44 female controls. About 50% of test and control animals survived 24-33 months [The Working Group noted that the experimental dose level used was too low for carcinogenic evaluation].

Levy & Clack (1975) gave 3 groups, each consisting of 30 male CB hooded rats, weekly doses of cadmium sulphate (0.09, 0.18 and 0.35 mg/kg bw Cd) by stomach tube for 2 years, at which time the experiment was terminated. The control group consisted of 90 rats. There was no difference in tumour incidence between exposed animals and controls. No neoplastic changes were found in the prostate. Renal concentrations of cadmium were on an average 5 µg/g wet kidney tissue in the highest exposure group; this level is below the average for adult human beings.

(b) Inhalation and/or intratracheal administration

Rat: Studies with cadmium oxide and cadmium chloride fumes (Paterson, 1947) were of too limited a duration for any conclusion to be drawn on the reported absence of tumours.

(c) Subcutaneous and/or intramuscular administration

Mouse: Gunn et al. (1963) found that a single s.c. injection of 0.03 mmol/kg bw (5.5 mg/kg bw) cadmium chloride in 26 Charles River mice damaged the testicular vascular supply. The tissue regenerated, but 14 months later, when the animals were killed, 77% of the mice had interstitial-cell tumours of the testis. No local tumours developed after 14 months in 25 mice receiving the same dose of cadmium chloride plus 3 mmol/kg bw (658 mg/kg bw) of zinc acetate. No tumours developed in 25 controls.

Of 20 male stock CB mice given 11 weekly s.c. injections of 0.05 mg cadmium sulphate in water into the right flank, none developed local tumours, and the incidence of neoplasms at other sites did not exceed that in a control group. However, testicular atrophy and moderate interstitial-cell hyperplasia were observed in 2 of only 5 animals surviving for 16-24 months and in 4/12 dead at 16 months (Haddow et al., 1964; Roe et al., 1964).

Rat: Heath & Daniel (1964) produced malignant local tumours in 9/10 and 6/8 female hooded rats given i.m. injections of 14 or 28 mg cadmium powder, respectively, into the thigh muscle. The last animals without tumours were killed at 84 weeks. A high proportion of the tumours were rhabdomyosarcomas, but some were fibrosarcomas; in general, they were fairly well differentiated, but many metastasized. These findings were confirmed by Heath & Webb (1967).

Zinc powder failed to inhibit cadmium powder tumourigenesis when both compounds were given i.m. to 2 groups of 25 male and 25 female Fischer rats. Either 2 injections of 5 mg cadmium powder or 1 of 3 mg cadmium powder plus 12 of 5 mg zinc powder were given at monthly intervals. By one year, 12 females and 14 males in the cadmium group and 8 females and 14 males in the cadmium plus zinc group developed fibrosarcomas (Furst & Cassetta, 1972).

Gunn et al. (1963) found in 25 Wistar rats that a single s.c. injection of 0.03 mmol/kg bw (5.5 mg/kg bw) cadmium chloride caused testicular vascular damage. The tissue regenerated, and after 11 months, when the animals were killed, 68% of the rats had interstitial-cell tumours of the testis. No interstitial-cell tumours developed in 20 controls. Of 17 rats which received cadmium chloride plus zinc acetate, 2 (12%) developed tumours of the testis after 11 months, when they were killed.

Gunn *et al.* (1964) reported that after a single s.c. injection of 0.03 mmol/kg bw (5.5 mg/kg bw) cadmium chloride in the interscapular region, 9/22 Wistar rats developed local sarcomas, and 19/22 developed interstitial-cell tumours of the testis after 10 months. Zinc acetate, given as 3 s.c. injections of 1 mmol/kg bw (183.5 mg/kg bw), inhibited the development of both types of tumours induced by cadmium chloride; the resulting tumour incidences were 2/17 for sarcomas and 3/17 for interstitial-cell tumours. No interstitial-cell tumours or local sarcomas developed in 18 controls.

A single s.c. injection of 0.03 mmol/kg bw (5.5 mg/kg bw) cadmium chloride in the hip induced local spindle-cell sarcomas in 6/45 male Wistar rats (Knorre, 1970a,b) and interstitial-cell tumours of the testis in 10/25 male Wistar rats observed up to two years (Knorre, 1971). Sarcomas developed between 7 and 18 months after injection, and interstitial-cell tumours after 12 months. Skin atrophy, ulceration and local necroses were noted soon after administration of the agent. No interstitial-cell tumours or local sarcomas developed in 32 or 20 controls observed for 706 days.

Lucis *et al.* (1972) gave male Wistar rats single s.c. injections of 0.02-0.03 mmol/kg bw (3.7-5.5 mg/kg bw) cadmium chloride. Interstitial-cell tumours of the testis developed in 13/15 rats before 11 months, and 2 rats developed local fibrosarcomas.

An intense inflammatory reaction with ulceration of the overlying skin followed a single s.c. injection of 25 mg cadmium oxide into ten female rats, and 8/10 animals developed local tumours within one year post-injection. No local tumours developed in 10 controls given a s.c. injection of saline alone (Kazantzis & Hanbury, 1966).

Of 20 male albino CB rats given 10 weekly s.c. injections of 0.5 mg cadmium sulphate in water into the right flank, 14 developed local sarcomas within 20 months after the start of treatment. All showed testicular atrophy, and many showed interstitial-cell hyperplasia. Of 18 rats examined *post mortem* within 20 months after the start of treatment, 10 had interstitial-cell tumours of the testis. Castration changes were observed in the pituitaries. All treated animals were dead by 20 months. No interstitial-cell tumours were seen in 16 controls that had died by 22 months. Similar results were obtained with cadmium-precipitated rat ferritin (Haddow et al., 1964; Roe et al., 1964), but no local tumours were induced by cadmium-free ferritin (Roe et al., 1968).

Repeated weekly s.c. injections into alternate flanks to 3 groups of 25 CB hooded rats of 0.05, 0.1 or 0.2 mg cadmium sulphate (0.02-0.09 mg Cd) for two years failed to produce neoplastic changes in the prostate gland. The control group consisted of 75 animals. Concentrations of cadmium in liver and kidney in the highest exposure group were of the same magnitude as those seen in occupationally exposed human beings (Levy et al., 1973).

A single s.c. injection of 25 mg cadmium sulphide into the dorsal skin of 15 male Wistar rats elicited an acute inflammatory reaction by 24 hours and extensive local fibrosis by three months (Kazantzis & Hanbury, 1966). In another experiment, a single s.c. injection of 25 mg cadmium sulphide produced sarcomas in 6/10 female Wistar rats at 6-10 months post-injection, and in 6/26 male and female rats between 9-19 months after injection. All animals died or were killed by one year (Kazantzis, 1963; Kazantzis & Hanbury, 1966).

Of 14 male and female rats given a single i.m. dose of 50 mg cadmium sulphide into the thigh, 5 developed local sarcomas from 9-15 months after injection (Kazantzis & Hanbury, 1966).

(d) Other experimental systems

Two groups of 30 and 11 rats received 4 simultaneous injections of cadmium chloride as 0.0015 mmol (0.17 mg) Cd or as 0.003 mmol (0.34 mg) Cd into 4 different tissue sites (s.c., i.m., subperiosteal and liver, kidney, salivary gland or ventral prostate). Local pleomorphic sarcomas were observed in 3 rats of the first group 12-16 months later; and in the second group, tumours developed at two s.c., one i.m. and one subperiosteal mesenchymal mesodermal sites about 10 months post-injection (Gunn et al., 1967).

3.2 Other relevant biological data

(a) Experimental systems

Harrison et al. (1947) exposed dogs to cadmium chloride mists in a chamber and found a LC_{50} of 0.32 mg cadmium/l of air for a 30-minute exposure. Death in all cases was due primarily to pulmonary injury, but tissue analysis showed that much of the cadmium chloride migrated from the lungs and was distributed throughout the body. The highest concentrations were found in the kidneys.

The LD_{50}'s in mice, rats, guinea-pigs, rabbits, dogs and monkeys for inhaled arc-produced cadmium oxide fumes during exposures ranging from 10-30 minutes were <700, 500, about 3500, about 2500, 4000 and 15,000 min mg/m^3, respectively (Barrett et al., 1947). The authors found that retention of the cadmium oxide by the animals' lungs was constant and amounted on average to 11%. Some cadmium was found in other organs, but it appeared to have originated from the ingestion of cadmium trapped in the upper respiratory tract.

Emphysema has been produced experimentally in male rats exposed to cadmium chloride aerosols (0.1% solution) for 1 hour per day on 5-15 days (Snider et al., 1973).

It is well established that cadmium damages the testes of experimental animals (Gunn et al., 1965; Parizek, 1960). It was demonstrated in mice that pre-treatment with zinc reduces the incorporation of cadmium into the spermatids and that cadmium inhibits the incorporation of thymidine into spermatogonia. Thus, serial mating studies after i.p. injection of 1 mg/kg bw cadmium chloride (purity unknown) into male mice significantly reduced the embryonic litter size of untreated females fertilized 15-48 days after treatment (Lee & Dixon, 1973).

Rabbits given 1 to 8 s.c. injections of 9-18 mg/kg bw cadmium chloride showed destruction of testicular cells (spermatogenic and interstitial) within the 5-21 days of the experiment. Hyperaemia and interstitial haemorrhage also occurred, and the kidneys, spleen and liver were also affected (Cameron & Foster, 1963). One s.c. injection of 0.05 mmol/kg bw (9.2 mg/kg bw) cadmium chloride (purity not specified) into rabbits induced aspermia within four weeks. Little recovery took place during the 17 weeks following treatment (Paufler & Foote, 1969).

It has been shown in several experiments in rats that kidney tubular lesions occur when the concentration of cadmium in the renal cortex is about 200 µg/g wet weight. Some data indicate that effects may occur below that level (Friberg et al., 1974, 1975).

Hypertension has been produced in rats given cadmium in drinking-water (5 µg/ml Cd) for long periods of time (Kanisawa & Schroeder, 1969b; Schroeder, 1964; Schroeder & Vinton, 1962). Perry & Erlanger (1974) found significant increases in blood pressure in rats given 1, 2.5 and 5 µg/ml Cd for one year in their drinking-water but not in animals given higher doses (10-50 µg/ml Cd).

Typical symptoms of zinc deficiency appear in rats given a sufficient amount of zinc but with an equimolar amount of cadmium (Petering et al., 1971); a large dose of zinc salt prevents the toxic action of cadmium on the testes (Friberg et al., 1974).

In studies in mice using aerosols of cadmium compounds particles of less than 2 µ were found in the lungs. With cadmium chloride, cadmium was found in the liver and kidneys; cadmium sulphide remained in the lungs (Potts et al., 1950). In many species, including mice, rats, guinea-pigs, rabbits, dogs and monkeys, about 5-25% of cadmium is retained after inhalation of cadmium compounds (Barrett et al., 1947; Potts et al., 1950).

Following single oral doses of ^{109}Cd or ^{115}Cd to mice (Nordberg, 1971a; Richmond et al., 1966; Suzuki et al., 1969), rats (Moore et al., 1973), monkeys (Friberg et al., 1974; Suzuki et al., 1974) and goats (Miller et al., 1968) only 1-3% of the cadmium was retained, and the absorption rate was probably of the same magnitude in the various species. In female mice, the biological half-life of a single oral dose of ^{109}cadmium was estimated to be 200 days (Richmond et al., 1966).

Moore et al. (1973) found in rats that after 4 hours' exposure to a ^{115}cadmium chloride aerosol (1.8 mg Cd/m^3) 9.7% of the inhaled amount was retained in the lungs. Data on cadmium concentrations in organs were not given.

In rats, absorbed cadmium is initially deposited in the liver but is slowly transferred to the kidneys (Gunn & Gould, 1957). Between 50 and 75% of the body burden occurs in liver and kidney; after long-term, low-level exposures the highest cadmium concentrations are found in kidney (Friberg et al., 1974).

Metallothionein has been found in the liver of cadmium-exposed mice and rabbits (Nordberg et al., 1971a, 1972), in the red-blood cells and plasma of mice (Nordberg et al., 1971b; Friberg et al., 1974) and in the duodenal mucosa of several species (Evans et al., 1970; Starcher, 1969). This low-molecular-weight protein is thought to play an important role in the transport of cadmium in the body. A single, high dose of cadmium partly bound to metallothionein had no effect on the testes in mice; the effect on the kidneys was more pronounced, and this may be explained by the fact that the cadmium-metallothionein is filtered through the glomeruli and reabsorbed by the kidney tubules (Nordberg, 1971b).

Cadmium chloride administered to rats by s.c. injection or directly into the liver is transported to the testes (Lucis et al., 1972).

^{109}Cadmium chloride given s.c. to rats appeared immediately in plasma and then disappeared rapidly; after six days only 2% of the dose was excreted in the faeces (Lucis et al., 1969). In rabbits, given 60 daily s.c. injections of cadmium sulphate, only about 1% of the daily dose was excreted in the urine each day (Friberg, 1952). In goats, dogs and rabbits given i.v. or s.c. injections, only a small percentage of the absorbed cadmium was excreted via the faeces (Axelsson & Piscator, 1966; Burch & Walsh, 1959; Miller et al., 1968).

Calcium deficiency increases tissue retention of cadmium in rats (Larsson & Piscator, 1971). That low calcium intakes will cause increased absorption and retention of cadmium has also been shown in rats by Washko & Cousins (1975). A low iron intake has also been shown to enhance the absorption of cadmium (Hamilton & Valberg, 1974).

Schroeder & Mitchener (1971) exposed mice for three generations to cadmium in drinking-water (10 µg/ml) and observed a reduction in litter size in breeding mice with loss of the strain after two generations and congenital abnormalities. Scharpf et al. (1972) produced teratogenic effects in rats by daily oral administration of 20 to 80 mg/kg bw cadmium chloride from day 6 to 19 of gestation. Some teratogenic effects may be explained by the interference of cadmium in maternal zinc metabolism.

In golden hamsters, i.v. injection of 2-4 mg/kg bw cadmium sulphate on the 8th day of gestation produced cleft lips and palates and other facial defects (Ferm & Carpenter, 1968). Teratogenic effects due to injected cadmium have also been seen in rats (Barr, 1973; Chernoff, 1973) and in mice (Ishizu et al., 1973).

(b) Man

Long-term exposure of man to large amounts of cadmium by inhalation or ingestion eventually causes renal tubular dysfunction (mainly proteinuria) (Holden, 1969; Piscator, 1962; Potts, 1965). The disturbances in mineral metabolism may eventually result in osteomalacia (Adams et al., 1969; Friberg et al., 1974).

Morgan (1970, 1971) observed a significant increase in renal, hepatic and blood cadmium concentrations in patients with bronchogenic carcinoma, a significant increase in hepatic cadmium concentration in patients with emphysema and a significant increase in renal and hepatic cadmium concentrations in patients with emphysema and bronchogenic carcinoma. The author, however, discounted the possibility that cadmium was responsible for these diseases.

Cadmium has been suspected of being a cause of hypertension in man, but so far no conclusive data have been presented to show such an effect (Friberg et al., 1974).

Only about 5% of ingested cadmium is absorbed (Rahola et al., 1972; Yamagata et al., 1974), and the amount eliminated in the faeces thus roughly corresponds to the ingested amount. Daily faecal excretion of cadmium has been reported to vary from 10 to 60 µg in non-exposed subjects (Essing et al., 1969; Tipton & Stewart, 1970; Tsuchiya, 1969; Wester, 1974).

Cadmium is stored, together with metallothionein, mainly in liver and kidneys; in the general population about one third of the body burden occurs in the kidneys (Friberg et al., 1974; Schroeder & Balassa, 1961).

The newborn is practically free from cadmium, but there is a steady rise in cadmium levels up to the 6th decade (Schroeder & Balassa, 1961). Average 'normal' levels in renal cortex at age 50 vary from about 15 to 30 µg/g wet weight; values of 50-125 µg/g have been reported in non-polluted areas in Japan (Friberg et al., 1974, 1975). Smokers generally have 5-100% higher renal concentrations of cadmium than do non-smokers (Lewis et al., 1972; Shuman et al., 1974).

It has been calculated that a daily intake of 88 µg would be necessary to achieve 50 µg/g wet weight in the renal cortex at age 50, assuming an absorption rate of 5%, a daily excretion of 0.01% of the body burden and that 10% of the daily absorbed dose is excreted rapidly each day (Friberg et al., 1974).

Urinary excretion of cadmium is low in the general population and is related to the body burden of cadmium (Friberg et al., 1974; Tsuchiya et al., 1976). It varies from less than 1 µg/day to about 3 µg/day in adults; smokers generally excrete more than do non-smokers (Piscator, 1976). The slow excretion corresponds to the long biological half-life of cadmium, which is estimated to be between 10 and 30 years (Elinder et al., 1976; Friberg et al., 1974; Tsuchiya & Sugita, 1971).

Intensive exposure in exposed workers may lead to a high excretion of cadmium; this probably mainly reflects recent exposure and is not accompanied by renal damage. With less intensive exposure excretion of cadmium in the urine is probably related to body burden. Renal tubular damage is thought to increase cadmium excretion (Friberg et al., 1974, 1975; Piscator, 1976).

Workers in a cadmium plant who were exposed to high levels of lead and cadmium were found to have a higher number of severe chromosome anomalies (chromatid exchanges, disturbances of spiralization, chromosome translocations, ring and dicentric chromosomes) but a lower total number of structural aberrations than rolling-mill workers exposed mostly to zinc but also to lower levels of lead and cadmium (Deknudt & Leonard, 1976).

Chromosome analyses were made in peripheral lymphocytes of 24 workers in a zinc smelting plant who had increased blood levels of cadmium and lead. The number of cells with structural chromosome aberrations was significantly greater than that in 15 controls; the mean in the exposed group was greater by a factor of 3 (1.35±0.99% in the exposed group *versus* 0.47±0.92% in the controls). The observed chromosome damage was mainly of the chromatid type (single breaks and exchanges) accompanied by acentric fragments. It was not reported whether exposure to other compounds such as arsenic also occurred (Bauchinger *et al.*, 1976).

An increased number of chromatid breaks and of aneuploid cells was observed in the lymphocytes of 12 patients with itai-itai disease who had had an excessive cadmium ingestion, as compared to that in the control population (Shiraishi, 1975). However, Bui *et al.* (1975) found no evidence that cadmium had induced chromosome aberrations in cultured lymphocytes from five cadmium-exposed Swedish workers and four Japanese itai-itai patients.

3.3 Observations in man

Reports from two industries have indicated a possible relationship between occupational exposure to cadmium oxide and prostate cancer. Potts (1965) reported a survey of 70 men exposed for 10 or more years to cadmium oxide dust in the production of alkaline batteries. Of the 8 deaths in this group, 3 were from prostate cancer and 2 from other forms of cancer. Kipling & Waterhouse (1967) reported results of an epidemiological study of 248 workers from the same factory with a previous history of at least one year's exposure to cadmium oxide. Prostate cancer was diagnosed in 4 cases, significantly more than the 0.58 cases expected on the basis of regional incidence rates. Three of the 4 cases are those referred to earlier by Potts (1965)[1]. Subsequently, no excess of any form of cancer was detected in three studies of men occupationally exposed to cadmium (Friberg *et al.*, 1974; Holden, 1969; Humperdinck, 1968), but each of these studies was of very small sample size or of insufficient time from the onset of exposure to permit a statistical evaluation of the carcinogenicity of cadmium.

---

[1]Personal communication from Dr M.D. Kipling

Lemen *et al.* (1976) reported on a cohort of 292 smelter workers with at least 2 years' exposure to cadmium oxide dust and fumes. Four deaths from prostate cancer were observed, while 1.15 would have been expected to have occurred in the total cohort. Although the risk of prostate cancer among the total study cohort was not significantly excessive, when further consideration was given to the time interval since the onset of exposure, a significantly increased risk of prostate cancer was demonstrated (4 observed *versus* 0.89 expected) 20 years following the onset of cadmium exposure. The authors also reported a significant excess of respiratory tract cancer: they observed 12 deaths where only 5.11 were expected [Data on smoking habits were not given].

4. Comments on Data Reported and Evaluation

4.1 Animal data

Single or repeated subcutaneous injections of several inorganic cadmium compounds (cadmium chloride, sulphate, sulphide and oxide) result in the development of local sarcomas in rats. Local tumours were also produced in rats by intramuscular injection of cadmium powder and cadmium sulphide.

Interstitial-cell tumours of the testis were observed following testicular atrophy in rats and mice given subcutaneous injections of soluble cadmium salts (cadmium sulphate and cadmium chloride). The pituitary glands of these animals showed castration changes.

Oral studies in mice and rats were inadequate for evaluation. No adequate long-term inhalation studies of carcinogenicity were available to the Working Group.

4.2 Human data

Available studies indicate that occupational exposure to cadmium in some form (possibly the oxide) increases the risk of prostate cancer in man. In addition, one of these studies suggests an increased risk of respiratory tract cancer.

5. References

Adams, R.G., Harrison, J.F. & Scott, P. (1969) The development of cadmium-induced proteinuria, impaired renal function and osteomalacia in alkaline battery workers. Quart. J. Med., 38, 425-443

Axelsson, B. & Piscator, M. (1966) Renal damage after prolonged exposure to cadmium. Arch. environm. Hlth, 12, 360-373

Banat, K., Förstner, U. & Müller, G. (1972) Schwermetalle in Sedimenten von Donau, Rhein, Ems, Weser und Elbe im Bereich der Bundesrepublik Deutschland. Naturwissenschaften, 59, 525-528

Barr, M., Jr (1973) The teratogenicity of cadmium chloride in two stocks of Wistar rats. Teratology, 7, 237-242

Barrett, H.M., Irwin, D.A. & Semmons, E. (1947) Studies on the toxicity of inhaled cadmium. I. The acute toxicity of cadmium oxide by inhalation. J. industr. Hyg., 29, 279-285

Bauchinger, M., Schmid, E., Einbrodt, H.J. & Dresp, J. (1976) Chromosome aberrations in lymphocytes after occupational lead and cadmium exposure. Mutation Res., 40, 57-62

Bui, T.-H., Lindsten, J. & Nordberg, G.F. (1975) Chromosome analysis of lymphocytes from cadmium workers and itai-itai patients. Environm. Res., 9, 187-195

Burch, G.E. & Walsh, J.J. (1959) The excretion and biologic decay rates of ^{115m}Cd with a consideration of space, mass and distribution in dogs. J. Lab. clin. Med., 54, 66-72

Bureau of National Affairs, Inc. (1975) National Wildlife Federation seeks defense phase-out of cadmium use. Environment Reporter, 29 August, pp. 703-704

Cameron, E. & Foster, C.L. (1963) Observations on the histological effects of sublethal doses of cadmium chloride in the rabbit. J. Anat., 97, 269-280

Chernoff, N. (1973) Teratogenic effects of cadmium in rats. Teratology, 8, 29-32

Church, F.W. (1947) A mixed color method for the determination of cadmium in air and biological samples by the use of dithizone. J. industr. Hyg. Toxicol., 29, 34-40

Deknudt, G. & Leonard, A. (1976) Cytogenetic investigations on leucocytes of workers from a cadmium plant. Mutation Res., 38, 112-113

Elinder, C.-G., Kjellström, T., Lind, B., Linnman, L. & Friberg, L. (1976) Cadmium in kidney cortex, liver and pancreas from Swedish autopsies. Arch. environm. Hlth (in press)

Essing, H.G., Schaller, K.H., Szadkowski, D. & Lehnert, G. (1969) Usuelle Cadmiumbelastung durch Nahrungsmittel und Getränke. Arch. Hyg. (München), 153, 490-494

Evans, G.W., Majors, P.F. & Cornatzer, W.E. (1970) Mechanisms for cadmium and zinc antagonism of copper metabolism. Biochem. biophys. Res. Commun., 40, 1142-1148

Fairbridge, R.W., ed. (1974) The Encyclopedia of Geochemistry and Environmental Sciences, Vol. IV A, New York, Van Nostrand-Reinhold, pp. 99-100

Ferm, V.H. & Carpenter, S.J. (1968) The relationship of cadmium and zinc in experimental mammalian teratogenesis. Lab. Invest., 18, 429-432

Flick, D.F., Kraybill, H.F. & Dimitroff, J.M. (1971) Toxic effects of cadmium: a review. Environm. Res., 4, 71-85

Friberg, L. (1950) Health hazards in the manufacture of alkaline accumulators. Acta med. scand. (Suppl. 240), 138, 1-71

Friberg, L. (1952) Further investigations on chronic cadmium poisoning. A study on rabbits with radioactive cadmium. Arch. industr. Hyg., 5, 30-36

Friberg, L., Piscator, M., Nordberg, G. & Kjellström, T. (1974) Cadmium in the Environment, 2nd ed., Cleveland, Ohio, Chemical Rubber Co.

Friberg, L., Kjellström, T., Nordberg, G. & Piscator, M. (1975) Cadmium in the Environment. III. A Toxicological and Epidemiological Appraisal, Washington DC, US Environmental Protection Agency

Fulkerson, W., Goeller, H.E., Gailar, J.S. & Copenhaver, E.D., eds (1973) Cadmium, The Dissipated Element, ORNL-NSF-EP-21, Oak Ridge, Tennessee, Oak Ridge National Laboratory

Furst, A. & Cassetta, D. (1972) Failure of zinc to negate cadmium carcinogenesis. Proc. Amer. Ass. Cancer Res., 13, 62

Furst, A. & Haro, R.T. (1969) A survey of metal carcinogenesis. Progr. exp. Tumor Res. (Basel), 12, 102-133

Greene, G.V. (1974) Cadmium compounds. In: Kirk, R.E. & Othmer, D.F., eds, Encyclopedia of Chemical Technology, 2nd ed., Vol. 3, New York, John Wiley & Sons, pp. 889-911

Gunn, S.A. & Gould, T.C. (1957) Selective accumulation of Cd^{115} by cortex of rat kidney. Proc. Soc. exp. Biol. (N.Y.), 96, 820-823

Gunn, S.A., Gould, T.C. & Anderson, W.A.D. (1963) Cadmium-induced interstitial-cell tumours in rats and mice and their prevention by zinc. J. nat. Cancer Inst., 31, 745-753

Gunn, S.A., Gould, T.C. & Anderson, W.A.D. (1964) Effect of zinc on cancerogenesis by cadmium. Proc. Soc. exp. Biol. (N.Y.), 115, 653-657

Gunn, S.A., Gould, T.C. & Anderson, W.A.D. (1965) Strain differences in susceptibility of mice and rats to cadmium-induced testicular damage. J. Reprod. Fertil., 10, 273-275

Gunn, S.A., Gould, T.C. & Anderson, W.A.D. (1967) Specific response of mesenchymal tissue to cancerogenesis by cadmium. Arch. Path., 83, 493-499

Haddow, A., Roe, F.J.C., Dukes, C.E. & Mitchley, B.C.V. (1964) Cadmium neoplasia: sarcomata at the site of injection of cadmium sulphate in rats and mice. Brit. J. Cancer, 18, 667-673

Haendler H.M. & Bernard, W.J. (1951) The reaction of fluorine with cadmium and some of its binary compounds. The crystal structure, density and melting-point of cadmium fluoride. J. Amer. chem. Soc., 73, 5218-5219

Hague, J.M. (1973) Preprint from the 1973 Bureau of Mines Minerals Yearbook, Cadmium, Washington DC, US Department of the Interior, pp. 1-8

Halbedel, H.S. (1966) Fluoboric acid and the fluoborates. In: Kirk, R.E. & Othmer, D.F., eds, Encyclopedia of Chemical Technology, 2nd ed., Vol. 9, New York, John Wiley & Sons, pp. 562-572

Hamilton, D.L. & Valberg, L.S. (1974) Relationship between cadmium and iron absorption. Amer. J. Physiol., 227, 1033-1037

Harada, A. (1973) Medical examination of workers in a cadmium pigment factory. Kankyo Hoken Rep. No. 24, September, p. 66

Harrison, H.E., Bunting, H., Ordway, N.K. & Albrink, W.S. (1947) The effects and treatment of inhalation of cadmium chloride aerosols in the dog. J. industr. Hyg., 29, 302-313

Heath, J.C. & Daniel, M.R. (1964) The production of malignant tumours by cadmium in the rat. Brit. J. Cancer, 18, 124-129

Heath, J.C. & Webb, M. (1967) Content and intracellular distribution of the inducing metal in the primary rhabdomyosarcomata induced in the rat by cobalt, nickel and cadmium. Brit. J. Cancer, 21, 768-779

Holden, H. (1969) Cadmium toxicology. Lancet, ii, 57

Humperdinck, K. (1968) Kadmium und Lungenkrebs. Med. Klin., 63, 948-951

IARC (1973) IARC Monographs on the Evaluation of Carcinogenic Risk of Chemicals to Man, Vol. 2, Some inorganic and organometallic compounds, Lyon, IARC, pp. 74-99

Ishizu, S., Minami, M., Suzuki, A., Yamada, M., Sato, M. & Yamamura, K. (1973) An experimental study on teratogenic effect of cadmium. Industr. Hlth (Kawasaki), 11, 127-139

Jache, A.W. & Cady, G.H. (1952) Solubility of fluorides of metals in liquid hydrogen fluoride. J. Phys. Chem., 56, 1106-1109

Kanisawa, M. & Schroeder, H.A. (1969a) Life term studies on the effect of trace elements on spontaneous tumors in mice and rats. Cancer Res., 29, 892-895

Kanisawa, M. & Schroeder, H.A. (1969b) Renal arteriolar changes in hypertensive rats given cadmium in drinking water. Exp. mol. Path., 10, 81-98

Kazantzis, G. (1963) Induction of sarcoma in the rat by cadmium sulphide pigment. Nature (Lond.), 198, 1213-1214

Kazantzis, G. & Hanbury, W.J. (1966) The induction of sarcoma in the rat by cadmium sulphide and by cadmium oxide. Brit. J. Cancer, 20, 190-199

Kipling, M.D. & Waterhouse, J.A.H. (1967) Cadmium and prostatic carcinoma. Lancet, i, 730-731

Kjellström, T., Lind, B., Linnman, L. & Nordberg, G. (1974a) A comparative study of the methods for cadmium analysis of grain with an application to pollution evaluation. Environm. Res., 8, 92-106

Kjellström, T., Tusuchiya, K., Tompkins, E., Takabatake, E., Lind, B. & Linnman, L. (1974b) A comparison of methods for analysis of cadmium in food and biological material. A cooperative study between Sweden, Japan and USA. In: Abstracts of papers presented at the CEE-EPA-WHO International Symposium on Recent Advances in the Assessment of the Health Effects of Environmental Pollution, Paris, 1974

Klein, A.K. & Wichmann, H.J. (1945) Report on cadmium. J. Ass. off. analyt. Chem., 28, 257-269

Knorre, von D. (1970a) Zur Induktion von Hautsarkomen bei der Albinoratte durch Kadmiumchlorid. Arch. Geschwulstforsch., 36, 119-126

Knorre, von D. (1970b) Örtliche Hautschädigungen an der Albinoratte in der Latenzperiode der Sarkomentwicklung nach Cadmiumchlorid-Injektion. Zbl. allg. Path., 113, 192-197

Knorre, von D. (1971) Zur Induktion von Hodenzwischenzelltumoren an der Albinoratte durch Kadmiumchlorid. Arch. Geschwulstforsch., 38, 257-263

Lai, M.G. (1974) Evaluation of analytical techniques for the determination of trace elements in marine waters. Naval Ordinance Laboratory, AD-787077, 24 July, Washington DC, US Department of Commerce

Larsson, S.E. & Piscator, M. (1971) Effect of cadmium on skeletal tissue in normal and calcium-deficient rats. Israel J. med. Sci., 7, 495-498

Lee, I.P. & Dixon, R.L. (1973) Effects of cadmium on spermatogenesis studied by velocity sedimentation cell separation and serial mating. J. Pharmacol. exp. Ther., 187, 641-652

Lemen, R., Lee, J.S., Wagoner, J.K. & Blejer, H.P. (1976) Cancer mortality survey of workers exposed to cadmium. Ann. N.Y. Acad. Sci. (in press)

Levy, L.S. & Clack, J. (1975) Further studies on the effect of cadmium on the prostate gland. I. Absence of prostatic changes in rats given oral cadmium sulphate for two years. Ann. occup. Hyg., 17, 205-211

Levy, L.S., Roe, F.J.C., Malcolm, D., Kazantzis, G., Clack, J. & Platt, H.S. (1973) Absence of prostatic changes in rats exposed to cadmium. Ann. occup. Hyg., 16, 111-118

Levy, L.S., Clack, J. & Roe, F.J.C. (1975) Further studies on the effect of cadmium on the prostate gland. II. Absence of prostatic changes in mice given oral cadmium sulphate for eighteen months. Ann. occup. Hyg., 17, 213-220

Lewis, G.P., Jusko, W.J., Coughlin, L.L. & Hartz, S. (1972) Contribution of cigarette smoking to cadmium accumulation in man. Lancet, i, 291-292

Linnman, L., Andersson, A., Nilsson, K.O., Lind, B., Kjellström, T. & Friberg, L. (1973) Cadmium uptake by wheat from sewage sludge used as a plant nutrient source. Arch. environm. Hlth, 27, 45-47

Ljunggren, K., Sjoestrand, B., Johnels, A.G., Olsson, M., Otterlind, G. & Westermark, T. (1971) Activation analysis of mercury and other environmental pollutants in water and aquatic ecosystems. Nuclear Techniques in Environmental Pollution, IAEA-SM-142a/22, Vienna, International Atomic Energy Agency, pp. 373-405

Lucis, O.J., Lucis, R. & Aterman, K. (1972) Tumorigenesis by cadmium. Oncology, 26, 53-67

Lucis, O.J., Lynk, M.E. & Lucis, R. (1969) Turnover of cadmium-109 in rats. Arch. environm. Hlth, 18, 307-310

Lyman, T., ed. (1961) Metals Handbook, 8th ed., Vol. 1, Novelty, Ohio, American Society for Metals, p.1199

Miller, W.J., Blackmon, D.M. & Martin, Y.G. (1968) ^{109}Cadmium absorption, excretion and tissue distribution following single tracer oral and intravenous doses in young goats. J. Dairy Sci., 51, 1836-1839

Moore, W., Stara, J.F., Crooker, W.C., Malanchuk, M. & Iltis, R. (1973) Comparison of ^{115m} cadmium retention in rats following different routes of administration. Environm. Res., 6, 473-478

Morgan, J.M. (1970) Cadmium and zinc abnormalities in bronchogenic carcinoma. Cancer, 25, 1394-1398

Morgan, J.M. (1971) Tissue cadmium and zinc content in emphysema and bronchogenic carcinoma. J. chron. Dis., 24, 107-110

Nordberg, G.F. (1971a) Effects of NTA on the toxicity and turnover of cadmium. Report to the Research Council, Stockholm, National Environment Protection Board

Nordberg, G.F. (1971b) Effects of acute and chronic cadmium exposure on the testicles of mice with special reference to protective effects of metallothionein. Environm. Physiol., 1, 171-187

Nordberg, G.F., Piscator, M. & Lind, B. (1971a) Distribution of cadmium among protein fractions of mouse liver. Acta pharmacol. (Khb.), 29, 456-470

Nordberg, G.F., Piscator, M. & Nordberg, M. (1971b) On the distribution of cadmium in blood. Acta pharmacol. (Khb.), 30, 289-295

Nordberg, G.F., Nordberg, M., Piscator, M. & Vesterberg, O. (1972) Separation of two forms of rabbit metallothionein by isoelectric focusing. Biochem. J., 126, 491-498

Oelschlaeger, W. & Bestenlehner, L. (1975) Bestimmung von Cadmium in biologischen und anderen Materialien mit Hilfe der AAS. Mitt. Landwirtsch. Forsch. (in press)

Organization for Economic Cooperation and Development (1975) Cadmium and the Environment: Toxicity, Economy, Control, Paris

Parizek, J. (1960) Sterilization of the male by cadmium salts. J. Reprod. Fertil., 1, 294-309

Pascal, P., ed. (1959) Nouveau Traité de Chimie Minérale, Vol. V, Paris, Masson, pp. 349-378

Paterson, J.C. (1947) Studies on the toxicity of inhaled cadmium. III. The pathology of cadmium smoke poisoning in man and in experimental animals. J. industr. Hyg., 29, 294-301

Paufler, S.K. & Foote, R.H. (1969) Effect of triethylenemelamine (TEM) and cadmium chloride on spermatogenesis in rabbits. J. Reprod. Fertil., 19, 309-319

Perry, H.M. & Erlanger, M.W. (1974) Metal-induced hypertension following chronic feeding of low doses of cadmium and mercury. J. Lab. clin. Med., 83, 541-547

Petering, H., Johnson, M.A. & Stemmer, K.L. (1971) Studies of zinc metabolism in the rat. I. Dose-response effects of cadmium. Arch. environm. Hlth, 23, 93-101

Petrovic, D. & Kalember, P. (1969) Occupational exposure to cadmium during the manufacture of miners' lamps and alkali accumulators. Arhiv hig. rada Toksikol. (Zagreb), 20, 187-197

Petrovic, D., Kalember, R. & Davidovic, M. (1968) Lesions caused by cadmium during the production of alkaline dry batteries. Vojnosanit. pregled (Belgrade), 25, 381-384

Piscator, M. (1962) Proteinuria in chronic cadmium poisoning. I. An electrophoretic and chemical study of urinary and serum proteins from workers with chronic cadmium poisoning. Arch. environm. Hlth, 4, 607-621

Piscator, M. (1976) Cadmium toxicity - industrial and environmental experience. In: Proceedings of the 17th International Congress on Occupational Health (in press)

Piscator, M., Adamsson, E., Elinder, C.-G., Pettersson, B. & Steninger, P. (1976) Studies on cadmium-exposed women. Abstracts, 18th International Congress on Occupational Health, Brighton, September 14-19 (in press)

Potts, A.M., Simon, F.P., Tobias, J.M., Postel, S., Swift, M.N., Patt, H.M. & Gerard, R.W. (1950) Distribution and fate of cadmium in the animal body. Arch. industr. Hyg., 2, 175-188

Potts, C.L. (1965) Cadmium proteinuria - the health of battery workers exposed to cadmium oxide dust. Ann. occup. Hyg., 8, 55-61

Rahola, T., Aaran, R.K. & Miettinen, J.K. (1972) Half-time studies of mercury and cadmium by whole-body counting. In: Assessment of radioactive contamination in man. Symposium on assessment of radioactive organ and body burdens, Stockholm, 1971, International Atomic Energy Agency Proceedings Series, New York, Unipub, pp. 553-562

Richmond, C.R., Findlay, J.S. & London, J.E. (1966) Whole-body retention of ^{109}cadmium by mice following oral, intraperitoneal and intravenous administration. US Atomic Energy Commission, University of California, Los Alamos Science Laboratory, LA-3610-MS, p. 195

Roe, F.J.C., Dukes, C.E., Cameron, K.M., Pugh, R.C.B. & Mitchley, B.C.V. (1964) Cadmium neoplasia: testicular atrophy and Leydig cell hyperplasia and neoplasia in rats and mice following subcutaneous injection of cadmium salts. Brit. J. Cancer, 18, 674-681

Roe, F.J.C., Carter, R.L., Dukes, C.E. & Mitchley, B.C.V. (1968) Non-carcinogenicity of cadmium-free ferritin. Brit. J. Cancer, 22, 517-520

Scharpf, L.G., Jr, Hill, I.D., Wright, P.L., Plank, J.B., Keplinger, M.L. & Calandra, J.C. (1972) Effect of sodium nitrilotriacetate on the toxicity, teratogenicity and tissue distribution of cadmium. Nature (Lond.), 239, 231-234

Schindler, C.P. (1967) Heterogeneous equilibria involving oxides, hydroxides, carbonates and hydroxide carbonates. In: Equilibrium Concepts in Natural Water Systems, Advances in Chemistry Series, No. 67, Washington DC, American Chemical Society, pp. 196-221

Schroeder, H.A. (1964) Cadmium hypertension in rats. Amer. J. Physiol., 207, 62-66

Schroeder, H.A. & Balassa, J.J. (1961) Abnormal trace metals in man: cadmium. J. chron. Dis., 14, 236-257

Schroeder, H.A. & Balassa, J.J. (1963) Cadmium: uptake by vegetables from superphosphate in soil. Science, 140, 819-820

Schroeder, H.A. & Mitchener, M. (1971) Toxic effects of trace elements on the reproduction of mice and rats. Arch. environm. Hlth, 23, 102-106

Schroeder, H.A. & Vinton, W.H. (1962) Hypertension induced in rats by small doses of cadmium. Amer. J. Physiol., 202, 515-518

Schroeder, H.A., Balassa, J.J. & Vinton, W.H., Jr (1964) Chromium, lead, cadmium, nickel and titanium in mice: effect on mortality, tumours and tissue levels. J. Nutr., 83, 239-250

Schroeder, H.A., Balassa, J.J. & Vinton, W.H., Jr (1965) Chromium, cadmium and lead in rats: effects on life span, tumors and tissue levels. J. Nutr., 86, 51-66

Shiraishi, Y. (1975) Cytogenetic studies in 12 patients with itai-itai disease. Humangenetik, 27, 31-44

Shuman, M.S., Voors, A.W. & Gallagher, P.N. (1974) Contribution of cigarette smoking to cadmium accumulation in man. Bull. environm. Contam. Toxicol., 12, 570-576

Sneed, M.C. & Brasted, R.C. (1955) Comprehensive Inorganic Chemistry, Vol. 4, New York, Van Nostrand, pp. 64-90

Snider, G.L., Hayes, J.A., Korthy, A.L. & Lewis, G.P. (1973) Centrilobular emphysema experimentally induced by cadmium chloride aerosol. Amer. Rev. resp. Dis., 108, 40-48

Stacey, M., Tatlow, J.C. & Sharpe, A.G., eds (1960) Advances in Fluorine Chemistry, Vol. 1, London, Butterworths Scientific Publications, pp. 88-89

Starcher, B.C. (1969) Studies on the mechanism of copper absorption in the chick. J. Nutr., 97, 321-326

Stecher, P.G., ed. (1968) The Merck Index, 8th ed., Rahway, NJ, Merck & Co., p. 186

Sunderman, F.W., Jr (1971) Metal carcinogenesis in experimental animals. Fd Cosmet. Toxicol., 9, 105-120

Sunderman, F.W., Jr (1976) Metal carcinogenesis. In: Goyer, R.A. & Mehlman, M.A., eds, Advances in Modern Toxicology, Chap. 3, Washington DC, Hemisphere Publishing Corp. (in press)

Suzuki, S., Taguchi, T. & Yokohashi, G. (1969) Dietary factors influencing upon the retention rate of orally administered $^{115m}CdCl_2$ in mice with special reference to calcium and protein concentrations in diet. Jap. J. industr. Hlth (Kawasaki), 7, 155-162

Suzuki, S., Taguchi, T. & Yokohashi, G. (1974) Gastrointestinal absorption and tissue distribution of cadmium after single oral exposure to monkeys. In: Proceedings of the 47th Annual Meeting of the Japanese Association of Industrial Health, Nagoya, March 29, pp. 120-121

Szadkowski, D., Schultze, H., Schaller, K.-H. & Lehnert, G. (1969) Zur ökologischen Bedeutung des Schwermetallgehaltes von Zigaretten. Blei-, Cadmium- und Nickelanalysen des Tabaks sowie der Gas- und Partikelphase. Arch. Hyg., 153, 1-8

Tarasenko, N.Y. & Vorobjeva, R.S. (1972) Hygienic problems connected with the cadmium use. Vestnik Akad. Med. Nauk SSR, 28, 37-43

Teworte, W. (1973) Blei, Zink, Cadmium - Gewinnung, Einsatz und Emissionen. Staub-Reinh. Luft, 33, 422-431

Teworte, W. (1975) Lead, zinc, cadmium - production, use and emissions. In: Heavy Metals as Air Pollutants. Lead, Zinc and Cadmium, Proceedings of the Colloquium held in Düsseldorf, 1973, VDI-Ber. 203, Düsseldorf, VDI-Verlag GmbH, pp. 5-15

Tipton, I.H. & Stewart, P.L. (1970) Patterns of elemental excretion in long-term balance studies. US Atomic Energy Commission Hlth Phys. Ann. Progr. Rep., July 31 1969, ORNL-4446, pp. 303-304

Tipton, I.H., Cook, M.J., Steiner, R.L., Boyes, C.A., Perry, H.M., Jr & Schroeder, H.A. (1963) Trace elements in human tissue. I. Methods. Hlth Phys., 9, 89-101

Tsuchiya, K. (1969) Causation of ouch-ouch disease. An introductory review. I. Nature of the disease. Keijo J. Med., 18, 181-194

Tsuchiya, K. & Sugita, M. (1971) A mathematical model for deriving the biological half-life of a chemical. Nord. hyg. T., 53, 105-110

Tsuchiya, K., Seki, Y. & Sugita, M. (1976) Organ and tissue cadmium concentrations of cadavers from accidental death. In: Proceedings of the 17th International Congress on Occupational Health (in press)

US Bureau of Mines (1970) Mineral Facts and Problems, Bulletin 650, Washington DC, US Department of the Interior, pp. 515-526

US Bureau of Mines (1975) Minerals in the US Economy, General Publication, 1975:3, Washington DC, US Department of the Interior, p. 17

US Environmental Protection Agency (1975) Scientific and Technical Assessment Report on Cadmium, EPA-600/6-75-003, March, Program Element 1AA001, Washington DC

Walker, R. (1974) Use and production of cadmium electrodeposits. Metal Finish., 72, 59-64

Washko, P.W. & Cousins, R.J. (1975) Effect of low dietary calcium on chronic cadmium toxicity in rats. Nutr. Rep. Intern., 11, 113-127

Weast, R.C., ed. (1975) CRC Handbook of Chemistry and Physics, 56th ed., Cleveland, Ohio, Chemical Rubber Co.

Wester, P.O. (1974) Trace element balances in relation to variation in calcium intake. Atherosclerosis, 20, 207-215

Whitnack, G.C. & Sasselli, R. (1969) Application of anodic-stripping voltametry to the determination of some trace elements in sea water. Analyt. chim. acta, 47, 267-274

WHO (1972) Sixteenth Report of the Joint FAO/WHO Expert Committee on Food Additives. Evaluation of mercury, lead, cadmium and the food additives amaranth, diethylpyrocarbonate and octyl gallate. WHO Food Add. Series, No. 4, pp. 51-59

Yamagata, N. & Shigematsu, I. (1970) Cadmium pollution in perspective. Bull. Inst. Publ. Hlth (Tokyo), 19, 1-27

Yamagata, N., Iwashima, K. & Nagai, T. (1974) Absorption of cadmium in the digestive tract of normal persons. In: Materials of the Research Meeting Concerning Cadmium Poisoning, Japanese Association of Public Health, March 16, Kankyo Hoken Rep. No. 31, pp. 84-85

NICKEL AND NICKEL COMPOUNDS*

Nickel and nickel compounds were first considered by an IARC Working Group in 1972 (IARC, 1973). Since that time new data have become available, and these are included in the present monograph and have been taken into consideration in the evaluation.

1. Chemical and Physical Data

1.1 Synonyms and formulae

Table I

(Chemical Abstracts names are underlined.)

Chemical Name	Chem. Abstr. Reg. Serial No.	Synonyms	Formula
Nickel	7440-02-0	Carbonyl nickel powder; C.I. No. 77775	Ni
Nickel acetate	373-02-4	Acetic acid, nickel (2+) salt; nickel (II) acetate; nickelous acetate	$Ni(COOCH_3)_2$
Nickel acetate tetrahydrate	6018-89-9	Acetic acid, nickel (2+) salt, tetrahydrate; nickel (II) acetate tetrahydrate; nickelous acetate tetrahydrate	$Ni(COOCH_3)_2 \cdot 4H_2O$
Nickel ammonium sulphate	15699-18-0	Sulphuric acid, ammonium nickel (2+) (2:2:1)	$Ni(NH_4)_2(SO_4)_2$
	51287-85-5	Sulphuric acid, ammonium nickel (2+) (1:2:1)	$Ni(NH_4)_2SO_4$
	25749-08-0	Sulphuric acid, ammonium nickel (2+) (3:2:2)	$Ni_2(NH_4)_2(SO_4)_3$

*Considered by the Working Group, December 1975

Nickel carbonate	3333-67-3	Carbonic acid, nickel (2+) salt; C.I. No. 77779; nickel (II) carbonate; nickelous carbonate	$NiCO_3$
Nickel carbonate, basic	39380-74-0	Nickel (2+) salt (1:1), mixture with nickel hydroxide [$Ni(OH)_2$] hydrate	$2NiCO_3 \cdot 3Ni(OH)_2 \cdot 4$
	1271-28-9	Zaratite	$NiCO_3 \cdot 2Ni(OH)_2 \cdot 4H$
Nickel carbonyl	13463-39-3	Nickel tetracarbonyl	$Ni(CO)_4$
Nickel chloride	7718-54-9	Nickel (II) chloride; nickel dichloride; nickelous chloride	$NiCl_2$
Nickel fluoborate	15684-36-3	Borate (1-) tetrafluoro-, nickel (2+); fluoboric acid, nickel (II) salt	$Ni(BF_4)_2 \cdot 6H_2O$
Nickel fluoride	10028-18-9	Nickel difluoride; nickel (II) fluoride; nickelous fluoride	NiF_2
Nickel hydroxide	12054-48-7	Nickel (II) hydroxide; nickelous hydroxide	$Ni(OH)_2$
	12125-56-3	Nickel (III) hydroxide Nickelic hydroxide	$Ni(OH)_3$ $NiO \cdot nH_2O$
Nickel iron sulphide	53809-87-3	Iron nickel sulphide; violarite	Ni_2FeS_4
Nickel mono-sulphide	16812-54-7	Nickel sulphide[1]	NiS
Nickel nitrate	21659-66-5	Nickel (II) nitrate; nickelous nitrate; nitric acid, nickel (2+) salt	$Ni(NO_3)_2$
Nickelocene	1271-28-9	Bis(η^5-2,4-cyclopenta-dien-1-yl)nickel; di-π-cyclopentadienyl-nickel	$(C_5H_5)_2Ni$

---

[1]This name is also used for nickel subsulphide; there is considerable confusion in the published literature between these two substances and other nickel sulphides (e.g., Ni_4S_3, Ni_2S, NiS_2).

Nickel oxide	1213-99-1	Green nickel oxide; nickel monoxide; nickelous oxide; nickel (II) oxide; nickel protoxide	NiO
	1314-06-3	Black nickel oxide; nickelic oxide; nickel (III) oxide; nickel sesquioxide; nickel trioxide	Ni_2O_3
Nickel subsulphide	12035-72-2	Heazlewoodite; nickel sulphide[1]	Ni_3S_2
Nickel sulphamate	13770-89-3	Nickel (II) sulphamate; sulphamic acid, nickel (2+) salt (2:1)	$Ni(SO_3NH_2)_2$
Nickel sulphate	7786-81-4	Nickelous sulphate; nickel (II) sulphate; sulphuric acid, nickel (2+) salt	$NiSO_4$

1.2 Chemical and physical properties

Physical properties of the nickel compounds considered in this monograph are given, when available, in Table II. Additional information on solubility is given below.

Nickel metal - soluble in dilute nitric acid and slightly soluble in hydrochloric and sulphuric acids (Weast, 1975). The solubility of metallic nickel in tissue and body fluids has been discussed by Weinzierl & Webb (1972).

Nickel acetate - soluble in acetic acid (12.4 mol. % at 30°C) (Stephen & Stephen, 1963)

Nickel ammonium sulphate - soluble in water (6.10 wt % at 20°C) (Stephen & Stephen, 1963); insoluble in ethanol

---

[1]This name is also used for nickel monosulphide; there is considerable confusion in the published literature between these two substances and other nickel sulphides (e.g., Ni_4S_3, Ni_2S, NiS_2).

Table II [a]

Chemical name	Atomic/mol. weight	Melting-point °C	Boiling-point °C	Crystal system	Density g/cm³
Nickel	58.71	1453	2732	face-centre cube [d]	8.90
Nickel acetate	176.80	dec.	16.6	prism	1.798
Nickel ammonium sulphate [b]	395			monoclinic	1.923 [d]
Nickel carbonate, basic [e]	376.24			cubic	
Nickel carbonyl	170.75	−25	43	liquid	1.32 (17°C)
Nickel chloride	129.62	1001	973 (subl.)		3.55
Nickel fluoborate [b]	232.31	dec.			
Nickel fluoride	96.71	1000 (subl.) (in HF)		tetragonal [a,c]	4.63 [a,c]
Nickel hydroxide	92.72	230 (dec.)			4.15
Nickel iron sulphide	301.27			isometric	5.3–5.65
Nickel monosulphide	90.77	797		trigonal	
Nickel nitrate [b]	290.81	56.7	136.7	monoclinic deliquescent	2.05
Nickelocene	188.90		130 (subl.)		
Nickel oxide NiO	74.71	1990		cubic	6.67
Ni₂O₃	165.42	600 (dec.) [d]			
Nickel subsulphide	240.26	790			5.82
Nickel sulphamate	252.90	500 (dec.)			
Nickel sulphate	154.78	848 (dec.)		cubic	3.68

[a] Data from Weast (1975) unless otherwise specified
[b] As the hexahydrate
[c] Haendler et al. (1952)
[d] Stecher (1968)
[e] Zaratite

Nickel carbonate, basic - insoluble in water, soluble in hot dilute hydrochloric acid and ammonium hydroxide (Weast, 1975)

Nickel carbonyl - very slightly miscible with water (0.016 g/100 ml at $9.8^{\circ}C$) (Weast, 1975); miscible with ethanol, benzene, chloroform, acetone and carbon tetrachloride

Nickel chloride - soluble in water (64.2 g/100 ml at $20^{\circ}C$ and 87.6 g/100 ml at $100^{\circ}C$) (Weast, 1975); soluble in ethylene glycol (16.2 wt % at $20^{\circ}C$), ethanol (9.13 wt % at $20^{\circ}C$) and hydrazine (0.8 g/100 ml at $20^{\circ}C$) (Stephen & Stephen, 1963)

Nickel fluoborate - very soluble in water and 95% ethanol; also soluble in ethanol/ether mixtures (Stacey *et al.*, 1960)

Nickel fluoride - slightly soluble in water (4 g/100 ml at $25^{\circ}C$) (Eméleus, 1950); soluble in acids, alkalis and ammonia (Weast, 1975)

Nickel hydroxide - soluble in aqueous ammonia; practically insoluble in water (0.00127 g/100 ml at $20^{\circ}C$) (Stephen & Stephen, 1963)

Nickel monosulphide - very slightly soluble in water (0.4 mg/100 ml at $18^{\circ}C$) (Weast, 1975)

Nickel nitrate - soluble in water (48.5 wt % at $20^{\circ}C$), in hydrazine (3 g/100 ml at $20^{\circ}C$) and in ethylene glycol (7.5 wt % at $20^{\circ}C$) (Stephen & Stephen, 1963)

Nickelocene - soluble in common organic solvents (Paulson, 1955)

Nickel oxide - nickel oxide (NiO) is practically insoluble in water (0.11 mg/100 ml at $20^{\circ}C$) (Blaszkiewicz, 1967). Nickel oxide (Ni_2O_3) is insoluble in water, very slightly soluble in cold acid, soluble in hot hydrochloric acid (with the evolution of chlorine) and soluble in hot sulphuric or nitric acid (with the evolution of oxygen) (Stecher, 1968).

Nickel subsulphide - insoluble in water and soluble in nitric acid (Weast, 1975). Its solubility in serum and in serum ultrafiltrate has been discussed by Sunderman *et al.* (1976).

Nickel sulphamate - soluble in water (Santmyers & Aarons, 1967)

<u>Nickel sulphate</u> - very soluble in water (27.3-27.7 wt % at 20°C); soluble in methanol (0.11 wt % at 35°C) and ethanol (0.02 wt % at 35°C) (Stephen & Stephen, 1963)

1.3 <u>Technical products and impurities</u>

Specifications from manufacturers indicate that impurities in nickel salts generally include some zinc, copper and iron. Typical compositions of nickel compounds and nickel metal have been described by Dean (1959).

2. Production, Use, Occurrence and Analysis

For important background information on this section, see preamble, p. 19.

Two reviews on nickel metal and alloys are available (Adamec & Kihlgren, 1967; Broache, 1970). A review of the chemistry of nickelocene is given by Barnett (1974).

2.1 <u>Production and use</u>

World mine production of nickel in 1971 was about 640 million kg, and in 1973 preliminary figures showed it to be about 660 million kg (Corrick, 1973). Table III gives the world production by country for 1973.

US demand for nickel increased from about 160 million kg in 1964 to 235 million kg in 1973 (US Bureau of Mines, 1975). In that year, nickel was used as follows: transportation, 20.9%; chemicals, 14.9%; electrical goods, 12.9%; fabricated metal products, 10%; miscellaneous uses, 9.7%; petroleum, 8.9%; construction, 8.9%; machinery, 6.9%; household appliances, 6.9% (US Bureau of Mines, 1975).

<u>Nickel metal</u> Nickel ingots and pellets are produced commercially by the electrolytic and Mond carbonyl processes. Its principal use is as an alloying additive in steel manufacture; it is also used in the production of coins, domestic utensils, monel metals and other alloys.

<u>Nickel powder</u> is produced commercially by the Mond process and its variations: nickel or nickel ore is reacted with carbon monoxide to produce nickel carbonyl gas, which is then decomposed by heat to give

Table III

World mine production of nickel[a] by country (Corrick, 1973)

Country[b]	Million kg
Australia (content of concentrate)	40
Brazil (content of ore)	≃ 3.1
Burma (content of speiss)	≃ 0.03
Canada[c]	243
Cuba (content of oxide and sulphide)	≃ 31
Dominican Republic	≃ 24
Finland (content of concentrate)	5.8
" (" " nickel sulphate)	≃ 0.2
Greece (recoverable content of ore)	12.6
Indonesia (content of ore)[d]	20.8
Morocco (content of nickel and cobalt ore)	≃ 0.3
New Caledonia (recoverable)[e]	99
Norway (content of concentrate)	≃ 0.4
Poland (content of ore)	≃ 2
Republic of South Africa	≃ 10.4
Rhodesia (content of concentrate)	≃ 12
United States (content of ore shipped)	16.6
USSR (content of ore)	≃136
Total	658

[a] As far as possible, this table represents mine production of nickel; where data relate to some more highly processed form, figures have been given to provide some indication of the magnitude of mine output; where only an estimate was available, this is indicated.

[b] In addition to the countries listed, Albania and the German Democratic Republic mine nickel, but available information is inadequate for reliable estimates of output levels to be made.

[c] Refined nickel and nickel content of oxides and salts produced, plus recoverable nickel in exported mattes and speiss

[d] Includes a small amount of cobalt not recovered separately

[e] Nickel-cobalt content of metallurgical plant products, plus recoverable nickel-cobalt in exported ores

pure, finely divided nickel. In another method of production, the nickel and cobalt contents of nickel oxide ores are recovered as carbonates, which are calcined to nickel oxide and reduced to nickel powder.

Many of the products made from nickel metal are also manufactured from finely divided nickel powder. It is also used as a hydrogenation catalyst.

Nickel acetate is produced commercially by reacting sodium acetate with a nickel sulphate solution. US consumption of all organic nickel salts in 1968 was estimated to be 227 thousand kg, almost all of which was nickel acetate.

It is used mainly as a mordant in the textile industry and to a minor extent as a hydrogenation catalyst.

Nickel ammonium sulphate is prepared by reacting nickel sulphate with ammonium sulphate (McMurdie *et al.*, 1971). It is used in electroplating, but to a lesser extent than is nickel sulphate (Antonsen & Springer, 1967).

Nickel carbonate   Only basic nickel carbonate ($2NiCO_3 \cdot 3Ni(OH)_2 \cdot 4H_2O$) is produced commercially. It is largely produced and consumed during the manufacturing of nickel oxide, nickel powder and nickel catalysts. Canada is the largest single producer of this material.

It has been estimated that 908 thousand kg of nickel salts other than nickel sulphate were consumed in the US in 1970; nickel carbonate probably accounted for most of these.

US consumption of basic nickel carbonate is largely in the production of nickel catalysts for use in organic chemical manufacture, petroleum refining and edible oil hardening. A high purity basic nickel carbonate is used in electronic components such as ferrites and thermistors. The total amount of nickel carbonate thus consumed is minor, but the number of individuals exposed could be quite high because of the large number of electronic component companies making and using ferrites and thermistors.

Nickel carbonyl is produced by the Mond process and its variations, as described above for nickel powder. Total annual production is estimated to be less than 6.8 million kg.

On a worldwide basis, the major uses of nickel carbonyl are as an intermediate product in the refining of nickel, in the manufacture of high purity nickel powder for powder metallurgy, in the fabrication of nickel and nickel alloy components and shapes and in the manufacture of catalysts. For these uses the carbonyl is contained within process equipment, with provisions to minimize human exposure in case of equipment failures. However, the facility with which it is made and converted into nickel has resulted in a large number of small-scale uses for the carbonyl, where exposure of personnel and venting to the atmosphere may constitute a hazard (e.g., vapour plating of nickel and depositing of nickel in semi-conductor manufacture).

Nickel chloride may be prepared from nickel oxide by chlorination or by reaction with hydrogen chloride (Antonsen & Springer, 1967). It is one of the principal nickel compounds used in electroplating (Antonsen & Springer, 1967).

Nickel fluoborate has been prepared from aqueous solution as the hexahydrate; it cannot be dehydrated without decomposition (Stacey *et al.*, 1960). Aqueous solutions are used directly in electroplating (Stacey *et al.*, 1960), and it is used as an electrolyte in high-speed plating (Antonsen & Springer, 1967).

Nickel fluoride may be prepared by the reaction of fluorine on finely divided nickel powder (Haendler *et al.*, 1952), by the reaction of anhydrous nickel chloride with fluorine or hydrogen fluoride, or by the fusion of nickel chloride with ammonium fluoride (Eleméus, 1950).

Nickel fluoride is used in battery cathodes (Cogley *et al.*, 1973).

Nickel hydroxide may be prepared from solutions of nickel salts by precipitation with alkaline hydroxides, but the product is usually contaminated by occluded or absorbed foreign salts. Pure nickel hydroxide can be prepared by electrolytic precipitation using nickel anodes (Antonsen & Springer, 1967).

It is used as a catalyst and in nickel-cadmium batteries (Antonsen & Springer, 1967).

Nickel monosulphide may be made by the direct fusion of nickel with sulphur (Antonsen & Springer, 1967); it is produced only in small quantities as a laboratory reagent.

Nickel nitrate is prepared by the reaction of nitric acid on nickel (Antonsen & Springer, 1967). It is used primarily as a catalyst and, to a lesser extent, in batteries.

Nickelocene may be prepared by the reaction of tetrapyridine nickel chloride and cyclopentadienyl sodium (Knox *et al.*, 1961) or by a simpler method using nickel chloride, cyclopentadiene and diethylamine (Watanabe *et al.*, 1965).

No evidence was found that nickelocene is produced in large quantities, but it is used as a laboratory reagent.

Nickel oxide is generally obtained by roasting refined nickel ores. Two partially reduced nickel oxide products, known as 'nickel oxide sinters', are produced commercially on a large scale; one contains 75% nickel and the other, 90%. Available data on nickel oxide products frequently combine information on nickel oxide powder and nickel oxide sinters.

Canada is the largest single producing country. In 1972, preliminary estimates of Canadian exports of nickel oxide were 33 million kg (Cajka, 1972). US imports of nickel oxide in 1973 (mostly from Canada) were 5.84 million kg (US Department of Commerce, 1974). In 1973, total US consumption of oxide powder and oxide sinter was reported to be 30 million kg (Corrick, 1973).

Most of the nickel oxide sinter produced is used in the manufacture of stainless and alloy steels.

Nickel subsulphide can be made by the direct fusion of nickel with sulphur (Antonsen & Springer, 1967); it is apparently not sold commercially.

Nickel sulphamate can be prepared by passing oxygen into a suspension of the powdered metal in aqueous sulphamic acid (Fischer, 1967). It is used in electroplating (Antonsen & Springer, 1967).

Nickel sulphate is produced commercially by dissolving nickel oxide in sulphuric acid and concentrating the solution to precipitate nickel sulphate heptahydrate, which on heating forms the commercial crystalline nickel sulphate hexahydrate (Antonsen & Springer, 1967).

Total US consumption in 1973 of nickel sulphate and other nickel salts was reported to be 3.3 million kg (Corrick, 1973). It is consumed as such in plating baths and also as an intermediate in the production of nickel ammonium sulphate and nickel carbonate, which are also used in nickel plating. It is used as an intermediate for depositing nickel carbonate on catalyst substrates and as the principal intermediate for the manufacture of organic nickel salts.

2.2 Occurrence

Nickel

Natural environment: Over 90% of the world's nickel is obtained from pentlandite $(FeNi)_9S_8$, a mineral invariably associated with large amounts of pyrrhotite and varying amounts of chalcopyrite. Secondary nickel minerals include garnierite and annabergite (Cornwall, 1966, 1973; Fairbridge, 1974).

Air: Reviews concerning air pollution by nickel have been made by Schroeder (1970) and by the CMBEEP (1975). Increasing use of nickel enhances the probability of its appearance in the atmosphere at nickel production plants. The average concentration of nickel in air samples collected from widely scattered locations in the US in 1964 and 1965 was 340 ng/m^3 (Falk, 1970). It constitutes 0.03% of the particulate matter suspended in the atmosphere (Sullivan, 1969). Nickel compounds, e.g., sulphides, oxides and carbonyl, enter the atmosphere as a result of the combustion of coal, diesel oil and fuel oil (Bowen, 1966; Natusch *et al.*, 1974).

Tobacco smoke: Traces of nickel are present in tobacco smoke (Szadkowski *et al.*, 1969). According to Sunderman & Sunderman (1961), at the time of their report six brands of American cigarettes contained an average of between 1.59 and 3.07 μg Ni per cigarette, and 20% of this found its way into the main-stream smoke.

Water: The concentration of nickel in various water samples ranged from 3-264 μg/l (CMBEEP, 1975).

Food: Nickel levels in various foods have been summarized by the CMBEEP (1975); concentrations of up to 6.5 µg/g in cereal food-stuffs, up to 2.6 µg/g in vegetables, up to 1.7 µg/g in fish and up to 7.6 µg/g in tea were recorded.

Animal tissues: Nickel levels in animal tissues were within the range of 0-5 µg/g wet weight (Schroeder et al., 1961); levels in various human tissues are summarized by the CMBEEP (1975).

Nickel carbonate occurs in nature as the mineral zaratite, $NiCO_3 \cdot 2Ni(OH)_2 \cdot 4H_2O$ (Cornwall, 1966). It is formed by the decomposition of nickel carbonyl in moist air and is a potential atmospheric and surface water pollutant.

Nickel carbonyl In addition to its use as a synthetic intermediate in plants producing nickel and nickel products, nickel carbonyl may be present wherever carbon monoxide contacts nickel and nickel alloys.

Nickel iron sulphide is found in nature as the mineral violarite, Ni_2FeS_4 (Cornwall, 1966). It is a secondary mineral formed from primary sulphides in the weathering zone by circulating ground water.

Nickel oxide The principal natural form of nickel oxide occurs in admixture with nickel sulphides in varying proportions in weathered ore. It is formed by the decomposition of nickel carbonyl in dry air.

Nickel subsulphide is found in nature as the mineral heazlewoodite, Ni_3S_2. It is not believed to be a significant atmospheric or water pollutant.

Nickel sulphate occurs as a minor mineral, morenosite, $NiSO_4 \cdot 7H_2O$ (Cornwall, 1966), formed in the weathering of primary nickel minerals. Because of its widespread use in plating baths, nickel sulphate may appear as a water pollutant in industrial areas where such baths are discarded or their parts washed after the plating operation.

2.3 Analysis

Several reviews on the analysis of elemental nickel have been published (CMBEEP, 1975; Lewis & Ott, 1970; Peshkova & Savostina, 1971). Atomic absorption spectrophotometry is one of the principal methods of analysis used for nickel in both air and water (Sachdev & West, 1970). The dimethylglyoxime method for colorimetric determination of traces of nickel was outlined by Sandell (1959). Gas chromatography has been used for the detection of nickel carbonyl in blood and breath (Sunderman *et al.*, 1968).

3. Biological Data Relevant to the Evaluation of Carcinogenic Risk to Man

Review articles on the biological properties and carcinogenicity of nickel compounds have been compiled by Sunderman (1973, 1976). The topic has also been reviewed by the Panel on Nickel of the US National Academy of Sciences (CMBEEP, 1975).

3.1 Carcinogenicity and related studies in animals

(a) Inhalation and/or intratracheal administration

Mouse: Hueper (1958) saw no abnormalities of the bronchial mucosa in 20 female C57BL mice exposed to an atmosphere containing 15 mg/m^3 of >99% pure nickel powder (majority of particles 4 μm or less diameter) for 6 hours per day on 4-5 days per week for up to 21 months. Two lymphosarcomas were observed; there was no unexposed control group, and all the mice were dead at 15 months.

Rat: Hueper (1958) exposed 50 male and 50 female Wistar rats and 60 female NIH Black rats to an atmosphere containing 15 mg/m^3 of >99% pure nickel powder (majority of particles 4 μm or less diameter) for 6 hours per day, 4-5 days per week for up to 21 months. Most of the animals (128/160) died before 15 months. In 15 of a total of 50 rats of both strains which were studied histologically, the lungs showed 'abnormal multicentric adenomatoid formation affecting the alveolar structures and atypical proliferations of the epithelial lining of the terminal bronchioli'. In some, but not all, rats 'subchronic inflammatory reactions' were associated with the adenomatoid formations; inflammatory changes and mucosal ulcers were found in the paranasal sinuses. The author regarded the adenomatoid lung lesions as benign neoplasms; there was no excess of neoplasms in other organs. No comparable unexposed control groups of rats were included in the experimental design.

Hueper & Payne (1962) observed no lung tumours in 120 rats, 46 of which survived for more than 18 months, following inhalation for 5-6 hours per day of 98.95% pure nickel powder (level unspecified) together with 20-35 ppm of a lung irritant (sulphur dioxide) and with powdered limestone, the latter being added to prevent the nickel particles from forming conglomerates.

Sunderman et al. (1957, 1959) exposed two groups of 64 and 32 male Wistar rats for 30 minutes thrice weekly by inhalation for 12 months to nickel carbonyl at concentrations of 0.03 and 0.06 mg/l, respectively. A further group of 80 rats was exposed once only to an atmosphere containing 0.25 mg/l nickel carbonyl, a level which approximates the LD_{50}. Animals were observed for up to 30 months after the first exposure, at which time all were dead. Inflammation of the lung was seen in all rats, and extensive squamous metaplasia of the bronchial epithelium in several; 4/9 rats surviving for 2 years developed neoplasms of the lung. One rat had a mixed adeno- and squamous-cell carcinoma with metastases to the kidney and mediastinum; a second rat had a similar but more anaplastic tumour; a third developed a squamous-cell carcinoma and a fourth, two papillary bronchial adenomas. The latter two animals were in the single exposure group. Of 41 control animals, only 3 survived 2 years, and none showed pulmonary tumours.

Starting with a group of 285 male Wistar rats, Sunderman & Donnelly (1965) observed a single pulmonary adenocarcinoma with metastases in 35 rats that survived 2 or more years after a single 30-minute inhalation of 0.6 mg/l nickel carbonyl (equivalent to the LD_{70} dose). A further group of 64 male Wistar rats was subjected to chronic inhalation of nickel carbonyl (0.03 mg/l for 30 minutes, thrice weekly until death): 1 rat had a pulmonary adenocarcinoma with metastases among 8 rats that survived 2 or more years after first exposure. No pulmonary carcinomas were found in 44 of a total of 70 male Wistar rats in 3 control groups that survived at least 2 years after the start of the experiments [Because of the rarity of spontaneous pulmonary malignancies in Wistar rats, the authors considered that the pulmonary adenocarcinomas were probably due to exposure to nickel carbonyl].

Kasprzak et al. (1973) administered nickel subsulphide (mean particle diameter, 10 µm) to 13 male Wistar rats as a single intratracheal injection of 5 mg/animal. The rats were observed for 15 months. No pulmonary tumours were found in these rats, although 4 had peribronchial adenomatoid proliferation; one rat developed a hepatoma. No untreated controls were used.

Ottolenghi et al. (1975) exposed 226 specific-pathogen-free male and female Fischer 344 rats to inhalation of nickel subsulphide (Ni_3S_2) for 6 hours a day on 5 days per week for 78 weeks, followed by observation for an additional 30 weeks. Seventy per cent of the particles of Ni_3S_2 were smaller than 1 µm, and 25% of the particles were between 1 and 1.5 µm in diameter. The concentration of Ni_3S_2 in the exposure chamber averaged 1 mg/m^3. For the controls, 241 rats were exposed to filtered room air for the same length of time. Rats exposed to Ni_3S_2 showed a significantly higher incidence of pulmonary hyperplastic and neoplastic lesions originating from the bronchial and bronchiolo-alveolar segments. The incidence of all lung tumours (benign and malignant) in the animals treated with Ni_3S_2 was 14%, compared to 1% in the controls ($P<0.01$). Fourteen malignant neoplasms of the lungs (10 adenocarcinomas, 3 squamous-cell carcinomas and 1 fibrosarcoma) were found in exposed rats; only one malignant neoplasm of the lung (an adenocarcinoma) was found in control rats. A small number (1.1%) of controls and a larger proportion (12%) of Ni_3S_2-treated rats displayed nodular hyperplasia and pheochromocytomas in adrenal medullae. Injection of hexachlorotetrafluorobutane, which induces lung infarction, did not increase the proportion of rats with pulmonary tumours, nor did it alter the types of pulmonary lesions found in exposed rats.

Hamster: Hueper & Payne (1962) saw no lung tumours in 100 male hamsters, 66 of which survived for more than 18 months, after simultaneous exposure to 98.95% pure nickel powder (level unspecified), 20-35 ppm (mg/kg) sulphur dioxide (acting as a lung irritant) and powdered limestone (1 part for 3-4 parts of nickel, to prevent nickel particles from forming conglomerates).

A group of 25 male and 25 female hamsters was given 30 weekly intratracheal injections of 0.2 ml of a suspension of 2 g nickel oxide (NiO) in 100 ml of 0.5% (w/v) gelatin in saline. The diameters of the particles of NiO ranged from 0.5 to 1 µm. A control group of 50 hamsters was treated similarly, except that carbon dust (nut-shell charcoal) was substituted for NiO. Only 1 tumour of the respiratory tract developed in the NiO-treated hamsters, compared with 4 tumours of the respiratory tract in the charcoal-treated hamsters; only 3 hamsters in each group survived 12 or more months after the end of treatment (Farrell & Davis, 1974).

Wehner (1974) and Wehner *et al.* (1975) exposed 51 male Syrian golden hamsters, 2 months of age, to chronic inhalation of nickel oxide (NiO) for 7 hours a day on 5 days per week for lifespan. The particle diameter of NiO dust was about 0.3 µm, and the mean atmospheric concentration of NiO was 52 µg/l. Four malignant tumours were detected at various sites in the NiO-treated hamsters, compared with 1 in 51 sham-treated controls. The authors concluded that there was no carcinogenic effect.

Guinea-pig: Hueper (1958) exposed 32 male and 10 female guinea-pigs of an inbred strain to an atmosphere containing 15 mg/m^3 of >99% pure nickel powder consisting of particles 4 µm or less in diameter for 6 hours a day on 4-5 days per week for up to 21 months. Only 23 animals survived for more than 12 months, and only 2 for more than 18 months. At death nearly all the animals were found to have 'abnormal multicentric adenomatoid formations affecting the alveolar structures and atypical proliferations of the epithelial lining of the terminal bronchioli'. One animal had an anaplastic intra-alveolar carcinoma; and another, with extensive pulmonary adenomatosis, showed a nodule in the abdominal cavity that was thought to be a metastasis from a pulmonary neoplasm, although no primary tumour was seen in the lung. No controls were used.

(b) Subcutaneous and/or intramuscular administration

Mouse: A group of 40 female Swiss mice received a single i.m. injection into each thigh muscle of 10 mg of a metallic dust taken from a flue at a nickel refinery. The dust contained 20% nickel sulphate, 57% nickel subsulphide and 6.3% nickel oxide and was administered as a suspension in penicillin G procaine. There were 36 survivors at 90 days; 23 sarcomas originating mainly in the striated muscle were formed at approximately one-third of the injection sites (average latent period, 11 months). Controls injected with penicillin G procaine developed no sarcomas (Gilman & Ruckerbauer, 1962).

When single doses of 5 mg nickel subsulphide or oxide were injected into one or both thigh muscles of Swiss or C3H mice, the percentages of sites with sarcomas were as follows: for nickel subsulphide, 53% in Swiss mice and 33% in C3H mice; for nickel oxide, 35% in Swiss mice and 23% in C3H mice. No such tumours were induced in Swiss mice similarly treated with cobalt oxide; no untreated controls were used (Gilman, 1962).

Rat: Heath & Daniel (1964) injected 28.3 mg pure nickel powder suspended in 0.4 ml fowl serum intramuscularly into the right thighs of 10 female hooded rats. Between 17 and 41 weeks after treatment, all of the animals developed local tumours; all were derived from striated muscle and most were well-differentiated. Metastases to pre-vertebral lymph nodes were seen in 3 rats. Previous findings in control rats had shown that local tumours were not produced following injections of fowl serum alone.

Furst & Schlauder (1971) gave repeated i.m. injections into the right thigh of nickel powder or nickelocene at monthly intervals to groups of 25 male and 25 female Fischer rats. With nickel powder, treatment consisted of 5 injections each of 5 mg in 0.2 ml trioctanoin: 38/50 rats developed fibrosarcomas within the 11 months of the treatment. In the same period, 18/50 rats given 12 injections of 12 mg nickelocene in 0.2 ml trioctanoin and 21/50 rats given 12 injections of 25 mg nickelocene in 0.2 ml trioctanoin developed fibrosarcomas. No fibrosarcomas developed in 50 control rats given 12 injections of trioctanoin.

Groups of 66 hooded and 20 Wistar rats were given i.m. injections into one or both thighs of 20 or 30 mg of a metallic dust taken from a flue at a nickel refinery. The dust contained 20% nickel sulphate, 57% nickel subsulphide and 6.3% nickel oxide and was administered as a suspension in penicillin G procaine. Sarcomas, most of them originating in striated muscle, were formed at approximately one-half of the injection sites in both strains after an average of only 5-6 months: 52 sarcomas occurred in hooded rats and 8 in Wistar rats. Control hooded rats injected with penicillin G procaine developed no sarcomas (Gilman & Ruckerbauer, 1962).

A similar result was obtained by injecting 20 mg of either nickel subsulphide (36 local tumours) or nickel oxide (26 local tumours) intramuscularly into one or both thighs; the mean latent periods of tumour induction were 150 and 302 days, respectively. However, no tumours were produced by i.m. injections of 5 mg nickel sulphate into both thighs of 32 Wistar rats observed for up to 603 days. No controls were used (Gilman, 1962).

Jasmin (1963, 1965) and Jasmin et al. (1963) investigated the effects of age, sex, castration and of an androgenic steroid upon the induction of sarcomas in Sprague-Dawley rats following single i.m. injections of 10 mg nickel subsulphide (Ni_3S_2) in 0.1 ml penicillin G suspension in the right gastrocnemius. In the initial experiment (Jasmin, 1963), 10 mg Ni_3S_2 alone were administered to one group of 15 female rats. In a second group of 10 female rats, 10 mg Ni_3S_2 were injected intramuscularly, followed by chronic daily s.c. injections of 0.5 mg methandrostenolone in saline. After 217 days sarcomas had developed at the site of Ni_3S_2 injection in 5/15 of the rats that had received Ni_3S_2 only and in 10/10 of the rats that had received Ni_3S_2 plus the steroid ($P<0.05$). In a second study (Jasmin et al., 1963), single i.m. injections of 10 mg Ni_3S_2 were administered to 14 female rats, 10 male rats and 10 castrated male rats. After 182 days, sarcomas had developed in 7/14 females, 3/10 males and only 1/10 castrated males. In a third study (Jasmin, 1965), single injections of 10 mg Ni_3S_2 were administered to 3 groups of 8, 10 and 14 male rats and to 3 groups of 10, 14 and 18 female rats at ages of 1, 2 and 3 months, respectively. After seven months local sarcomas had developed in 8/14, 7/10 and 3/8 rats in the 3 groups of males and in 4/10, 15/18 and 4/10 rats in the 3 groups of females. Jasmin (1965) concluded that maximum susceptibility to sarcoma induction after i.m. injection of Ni_3S_2 in male and female Sprague-Dawley rats occurred at 2 months of age. Jasmin (1963, 1965) and Jasmin et al. (1963) did not study untreated control rats or rats that received only an injection of the vehicle (penicillin G suspension) alone.

Daniel (1966) compared the responses of three different strains of male and female rats (hooded, Fischer and NIH Black) to the i.m. injection of 10 mg nickel subsulphide in 0.1 ml aqueous penicillin G procaine into each gastrocnemius muscle. Local tumours developed invariably in both legs of all 28 hooded rats and in one leg only of 14/27 NIH Black rats; more of the tumours in the hooded strain were well-differentiated rhabdomyosarcomas.

There were no controls. In another experiment, the early response (2-10 weeks) of Fischer rats was found to be more like that of the hooded strain than that of the NIH Black strain. Necrosis and abnormal myoblasts were features of the response of Fischer and hooded rats, and active phagocytosis of nickel subsulphide a feature of the response of NIH Black rats.

Maenza et al. (1971) administered a total of 20 mg nickel subsulphide (Ni_3S_2) in 1 ml of an aqueous suspension of penicillin G procaine to 30 male Fischer rats in two simultaneous bilaterial i.m. injections (10 mg Ni_3S_2/injection site). The Ni_3S_2 powder had a mean particle diameter of 2 μm. Thirty control rats were given bilateral injections of the vehicle alone. The rats were observed for 104 weeks. In the Ni_3S_2-treated group, sarcomas developed at at least one injection site in 30/30 rats, and sarcomas developed at both injection sites in 12/30 rats. No sarcomas occurred at either injection site in any of the 30 control rats. All of the Ni_3S_2 rats had died by 47 weeks after the injection, while all of the control rats survived until the end of the experiment. Eighty-one per cent of the primary sarcomas were classified as rhabdomyosarcomas, and distant metastases were found in 57% of the Ni_3S_2-treated rats.

Mason et al. (1971) and Mason (1972) administered nickel subsulphide to 160 Fischer rats, divided into four subgroups (A,B,C and D) of 40 rats each (20 males, 20 females). Rats in groups A and B received single s.c. injections of 10 and 3.3 mg, respectively, of Ni_3S_2 suspended in 0.1 ml aqueous penicillin G procaine. Rats in groups C and D received single i.m. injections of 10 and 3.3 mg Ni_3S_2 in the same vehicle, respectively. One group of 120 rats (60 males, 60 females) was given twice weekly injections of 0.25 ml saline solution for 52 weeks; a second group of 120 control rats (60 males, 60 females) was given no treatment. The study was terminated at 18 months, and the incidences of sarcomas at the site of injection of Ni_3S_2, predominately rhabdomyosarcomas, in groups A-D were 90, 95, 85 and 97%, respectively. No sarcomas were found in any of the control rats.

Sunderman et al. (1974) administered 2.5 mg nickel subsulphide to 40 male Fischer rats as a single i.m. injection in 0.5 ml penicillin G procain suspension into the thigh. The mean particle diamter of the Ni_3S_2 dust was 1.4 μm. A control group of 24 rats was given a single i.m. injection of the vehicle. Surviving rats were killed two years after the injection. Local sarcomas developed in 39/40 Ni_3S_2-treated rats and in 0/24 control rats. Thirteen of the 39 sarcomas (33%) were classified as rhabdomyosarcomas, and the remaining sarcomas were predominantly fibrosarcomas or undifferentiated sarcomas. Fifteen of the 39 sarcomas (38%) metastasized to distant sites, including the lungs, mediastinum, heart, liver, spleen, mesentery and para-aortic lymph nodes.

Sunderman *et al.* (1975, 1976) studied the dose-response relationship for induction of sarcomas in male Fischer rats after i.m. injection of nickel subsulphide in 0.5 ml penicillin G procaine suspension. Ni_3S_2 dust (mean particle diameter, 1.4 μm) was administered to 4 groups of 30 rats in doses of 0.63, 1.25, 2.5 and 5 mg, respectively. A control group of 60 rats was given an i.m. injection of the vehicle. Surviving rats were killed 2 years after the injection. Local sarcomas developed in 7/30 rats which received 0.63 Ni_3S_2, compared with sarcoma incidences of 23/30, 28/30 and 29/30 in rats that received dosages of 1.25, 2.5 and 5 mg Ni_3S_2, respectively. No local sarcomas occurred in any of the 60 control rats.

Sunderman & Maenza (1976) compared the carcinogenicities of nickel subsulphide, nickel monosulphide, nickel dust and partially converted matte (nickel iron sulphide) after i.m. administration to groups of 10 male Fischer rats at two dose levels. The mean particle diameters of the powders were all less than 2 μm; the powders were suspended in 0.5 ml aqueous penicillin G procaine. One control group of 20 Fischer rats was given an i.m. injection of the vehicle alone; two additional control groups of 10 Fischer rats each were given i.m. injections of iron dust at two dose levels. Surviving rats were killed 2 years after the injection. The results of the study are summarized in Table IV.

Numerous investigators have administered i.m. or s.c. injections of nickel or nickel subsulphide to rats in order to induce sarcomas, as a preliminary step in ultrastructural, cytogenetic, tissue cultural, biochemical, immunological or chemotherapeutic studies of the resulting tumours. Reviews by Sunderman (1973, 1976) contain tabulations of such investigations of nickel carcinogenesis in rats.

Hamster: Furst & Schlauder (1971) injected nickel powder or nickelocene intramuscularly at monthly intervals into groups of 25 male and 25 female hamsters. Nickel powder treatment consisted of 5 injections each of 5 mg in 0.2 ml trioctanoin; by 11 months after the first injection 2 males had developed fibrosarcomas. Of 50 controls given 9 i.m. injections of 0.2 ml trioctanoin, none developed fibrosarcomas. Of 50 hamsters given a single injection of 25 mg nickelocene in 0.2 ml trioctanoin, 29 survived for 11 months; of these, 4 developed fibrosarcomas. Of 50 hamsters given 8 injections of 5 mg nickelocene in 0.2 ml trioctanoin, none developed fibrosarcomas.

<u>Table IV</u>

Sarcoma induction after i.m. injection of metallic compounds in Fischer rats[a]

Compound	Dose		Local sarcoma incidence by 2 years
	mg/rat	μm-atom of metal/rat	
None[b]	0	0	0/20
Ni_3S_2	5.0	60	8/10[c]
	20.0	240	9/10[c]
NiS	5.6	60	0/10
	22.4	240	0/10
Ni	3.6	60	0/10
	14.4	240	2/10
Fe	3.5	60	0/10
	14.0	240	0/10
Ni_4FeS_4[d]	9.2	85 (Ni)	1/10
	36.8	340 (Ni)	8/10[c]

[a] Sunderman & Maenza (1976)

[b] Rats in this control group received a single i.m. injection of 0.5 ml of the vehicle (penicillin G procaine suspension).

[c] $P<0.001$ compared with controls (χ^2 test)

[d] Partially converted matte (54% Ni, 14% Fe, 32% S)

(c) Intravenous administration

Mouse: Hueper (1955) saw no neoplasms in response to 2 i.v. injections of 0.05 ml of a 0.005% suspension of nickel powder in 2.5% gelatin into the tail vein of 25 C57BL male mice, 19 of which lived for more than one year and 6 of which lived for more than 15 months. No controls were used.

Rat: Hueper (1955) gave 6 weekly injections of 0.5 ml/kg bw of a 0.5% suspension of nickel powder in physiological saline in the saphenous vein of 25 Wistar rats. The only neoplasms that could be attributed to treatment arose 7-8 months after the first injection in 7 rats near the site of injection (region of groin), where seepage of the injected material had occurred. Deposits of black powder in the lungs in 2 rats indicated that at least some of the injected material remained in the vein at the time of injection. No controls were used.

Lau $et\ al.$ (1972) injected 6 doses of 20 μl/kg bw nickel carbonyl (9 mg Ni/kg bw) into the tail vein at intervals of 2-4 weeks into male and female Sprague-Dawley rats. The animals were observed until death. Of 61 males and 60 females that survived the 6 injections, 19 (16%) developed malignant tumours, comprising 6 undifferentiated sarcomas at various sites, 3 fibrosarcomas at various sites, 1 liver carcinoma, 1 kidney carcinoma, 1 mammary carcinoma, 1 haemangioendothelioma, 1 undifferentiated leukaemia and 5 pulmonary lymphomas. Among 15 male and 32 female sham-injected controls, the only malignant tumours seen were 2 pulmonary lymphomas. The difference in incidences of malignant tumours between treated and control rats was statistically significant ($P<0.05$).

Rabbit: Hueper (1955) saw no neoplasms in 10 rabbits given 6 weekly injections of 0.5 ml/kg bw of a 1% suspension of nickel powder in 25% aqueous gelatin solution. Only 4 of the rabbits survived for more than 2 years. No effects were seen in 5 control rabbits observed up to 40 months.

(d) Other experimental systems

Intrapulmonary administration: Hueper & Payne (1962) introduced fine nickel powder (0.02 ml of a suspension of 0.2 g nickel/ml of 10% gelatin) directly into the lungs of 34 NIH Black rats by thoracotomy. All survivors were similarly treated 12 months later. Of 14 rats that lived for 18 or more months after the first treatment, one developed a sarcoma at the site of injection. No epithelial tumours of the lung were seen. No controls were used.

Intrapleural administration: Hueper (1955) saw no neoplasms attributable to treatment in 50 C57BL male mice, 37 of which survived for more than 12 months and 4 of which survived for more than 18 months, after a single injection of 0.02 ml of a 0.06% suspension of nickel powder in 2.5% gelatin-saline solution.

Hueper (1952) reported the formation of round-cell and spindle-cell tumours at the site of injection in 4/12 female Osborne-Mendel rats that died between 7 and 16 months after 5 monthly injections of 0.05 ml of a 12.5% (by volume) suspension of nickel powder in lanolin.

Furst et al. (1973) administered 5 monthly injections of 5 mg nickel powder in 0.2 ml saline to 5 male and 5 female Fischer rats. Twenty control rats (10 males, 10 females) were given 5 monthly injections of saline solution. Pleural mesotheliomas developed in 2/10 of the Ni-treated rats and in 0/20 controls.

Intramedullary injection into the femur: Hueper (1952) reported 1 squamous-cell carcinoma of a fistulous duct and 3 osteosarcomas at the site of injection in 4/17 female Osborne-Mendel rats surviving 7 months after an injection of 0.05 ml of a 12.5% (by volume) suspension of nickel powder in lanolin. This finding was not confirmed in a subsequent study (Hueper, 1955) in which 27/100 Wistar rats, 40 of which survived for more than 18 months, developed neoplasms at or near the site of injection of 0.1 ml of a 5% suspension of nickel powder in 20% gelatin-saline. Some animals received a second injection after 18 months. The author commented that there was usually some seepage of the nickel suspension from the marrow cavity into the periosteal tissue. Sixteen of the tumours were fibrosarcomas; 4 were rhabdomyosarcomas; 5 were thought to be neurogenic in origin; 1 was an angiosarcoma; and 1, a reticulum-cell sarcoma. Metastases were seen in 14/27 rats bearing injection-site tumours. In addition, 20 neoplasms were seen at sites remote from the injection site, but their occurrence was not considered to be causally related to nickel.

Hueper (1955) reported that 1/6 rabbits given 2 injections, 27 months apart, of 0.25 ml nickel powder in lanolin (12.5% nickel by volume) developed a metastasizing endosteal fibrosarcoma of the femur. Two rabbits given injections of lanolin alone did not develop local tumours.

Implantation: Gilman (1966) reported the occurrence of rhabdomyosarcomas in 2/45 and fibrosarcomas in 14/45 Swiss mice given a single i.m. implant of 5 mg nickel subsulphide; 5 rhabdomyosarcomas and 16 fibrosarcomas were seen in 50 Swiss mice similarly treated with nickel oxide. No controls were used.

Mitchell et al. (1960) implanted 4 nickel pellets (2 mm diameter) subdermally in each of 5 male and 5 female Wistar rats. Within 104 weeks after implantation of the nickel pellets, 3 males and 2 females had developed sarcomas around one pellet. In another group of rats that received similar implantations of pellets of a nickel-gallium alloy, sarcomas developed around one or more pellets in 9/10 rats. In contrast, no tumours occurred in 10 other groups of 10 rats each that received similar implants of pellets of various materials that have been used in dentistry, including fused porcelain, silver, silver amalgam, vitallium and copper.

Gilman & Herchen (1963) induced tumours in groups of 20 Fischer rats by the i.m. implantation into both gluteal regions of nickel subsulphide administered either as 10 mg of powder with particles of 2-4 μm diameter, 500 mg as 3-5 mm diameter fragments, 500 mg as single discs of 11 mm diameter, or as 10 mg of powder within a millipore diffusion chamber. Rhabdomyosarcomas arose in approximately 70% of implantation sites in all 4 groups. Several tumours gave rise to distant metastases. Only 1/19 control rats that received 2 implants each of empty diffusion chambers developed a tumour.

Herchen & Gilman (1964) implanted solid discs of compressed nickel subsulphide powder (measuring 8 x 1 mm and weighing approximately 250 mg) into the right gluteal regions of 120 inbred Fischer rats. The implants were removed from groups of ten rats after 2, 4, 8, 16, 32, 64, 128 and 256 days. Palpable local tumours arose in 4, 7 and 10 rats in the last three groups, respectively. For control purposes, similarly sized discs of ferric oxide were implanted into the left gluteal regions of the same animals: no local tumours arose at the sites of ferric oxide implants, irrespective of how long they remained *in situ*.

Payne (1964) compared the carcinogenicities of 9 nickel compounds (7 mg) of varying solubility by 3 surgical implantations of the compounds, formed into pellets with sheep fat, into the muscle (unspecified) of groups of 35 NIH Black rats. Pellets of sheep fat alone were similarly implanted in a control group of 35 rats. After 18 months, 12/35 rats implanted with nickel subsulphide, 6/35 rats implanted with nickel carbonate and 4/35 rats implanted with nickel oxide (NiO) had developed sarcomas at the site of implantation. Single sarcomas were observed with implantations of nickel sulphate and nickel acetate tetrahydrate. No tumours were observed at implantation sites in rats that received nickel chloride, nickel acetate, nickel ammonium sulphate or nickel oxide (Ni_2O_3) or in controls. The author concluded that the carcinogenicity of each compound was a reflection of its solubility and of the valence state of the nickel.

Gilman (1966) reported the induction of rhabdomyosarcomas in 9/17 and fibrosarcomas in 3/17 rats following the introduction (presumably into the thigh muscles) of millipore diffusion chambers containing 10 mg nickel subsulphide. This observation was taken to indicate that direct contact between metal particles and cells is not necessary for carcinogenesis. The same paper reported the induction of tumours at the site of implantation in 22/40 Wistar rats given nickel subsulphide and in 19/40 Wistar rats given nickel hydroxide but, in contrast, in 0/28 Wistar rats given nickel monosulphide. A dose-response relationship was found for nickel subsulphide and the induction of rhabdomyosarcomas in Fischer rats: 10 mg per site gave an 80% tumour incidence. No controls were used.

3.2 Other relevant biological data

Hackett & Sunderman (1969) reported that i.v. administration to rats of nickel carbonyl in LD_{50}-LD_{100} doses led to diffuse dilatation of the rough-surfaced endoplasmic reticulum and nucleolar fragmentation in hepatic cells. Sunderman (1967b) found that inhalation of nickel carbonyl inhibited phenothiazine induction of benzo[*a*]pyrene hydroxylase in the lung and liver of rats.

Swierenga (1970) reported that in tissue cultures of rat embryo muscle cells, nickel subsulphide profoundly inhibited glyceraldehyde-3-phosphate dehydrogenase activity, whereas nickel chloride and nickel sulphate cause only slight inhibition of this important glycolytic enzyme.

After acute or chronic exposure of rats to nickel carbonyl by inhalation, increases in nickel occur predominantly in the microsomal and supernatant fractions of lung and liver. After chronic exposure, increased amounts of nickel are also observed in nuclear and mitochondrial fractions of the lung (Sunderman & Sunderman, 1963).

Webb et al. (1972) studied the intracellular distribution of nickel in nickel-induced rhabdomyosarcomas in the rat and found that a major portion (70-90%) occurs within the nucleus. Furthermore, subfractionation indicated that an average of 53% (range 41-63%) of nuclear nickel is present in the nucleolar fraction. Nucleolar localization of nuclear nickel has also been observed by Webb & Weinzierl (1972) in mouse dermal fibroblasts grown *in vitro* in the presence of $^{63}Ni^{2+}$ complexes.

Sunderman et al. (1974) gave 5 groups of 10, 24 or 40 male Fischer rats single i.m. injections of 2.5 mg nickel subsulphide (Ni_3S_2) alone or in combination with equimolar amounts of aluminium, copper, chromium or manganese dusts. Rats in 5 control groups were treated identically, except that the Ni_3S_2 dust was omitted. After 24 months, the incidence of local sarcomas was 15/24 (63%) (P<0.001 *versus* Ni_3S_2 alone) in the group that received the combination of Ni_3S_2 and manganese dusts; incidences of 96 to 100% were seen in the groups that received Ni_3S_2 alone or in combination with aluminium, copper or chromium dusts. No local sarcomas occurred in the 106 rats in the 5 control groups. The finding that concurrent administration of manganese dust decreases tumourigenesis induced by i.m. injection of Ni_3S_2 in Fischer rats has been confirmed in other studies by Sunderman et al. (1975, 1976).

RNA derived from the lungs of rats exposed to nickel carbonyl showed abnormal physico-chemical properties (Sunderman, 1963). This compound inhibits the synthesis of hepatic RNA, as demonstrated by the inhibition of cortisone induction of hepatic tryptophan pyrrolase (Sunderman, 1967a), inhibition of ^{14}C-orotic acid incorporation *in vivo* into liver RNA

(Beach & Sunderman, 1969) and inhibition of DNA-dependent RNA-polymerase activity in hepatic nuclei (Sunderman, 1971; Witschi, 1972). Beach & Sunderman (1970) have shown that the inhibition of RNA synthesis persists after the disruption of hepatic nuclei, and they exclude the possibility that inhibition is due to impaired transport of RNA precursors across the nuclear membrane. Nickel carbonyl resembles actinomycin D in its differential effects upon hepatic synthesis of RNA (high inhibition) and proteins (low inhibition) and in its inhibitory effects on liver enzyme induction (Sunderman, 1971).

Basrur & Gilman (1967) and Swierenga & Basrur (1968) showed that addition of nickel subsulphide to cultured embryonic muscle cells inhibits mitotic activity and induces abnormal mitotic figures. Their findings suggest that nickel may interfere with gene replication and with the control of cell division. Olinici et al. (1973) reported the presence of marker chromosomes in two cell lines in tissue cultures of Ni-induced rhabdomyosarcomas. In both cell lines, chromosomal abnormalities persisted through many transplant generations.

Those nickel compounds which have been shown to be carcinogenic in experimental animals have not been tested for mutagenicity. Soluble nickel compounds (nickel chloride and sulphate) which have not produced tumours in experimental animals have likewise produced negative results in two mutagenicity tests (Buselmaier et al., 1972; Corbett et al., 1970).

3.3 Observations in man

Ten cases of cancer of the nasal cavities among workers in a nickel refinery in Clydach, Wales, were described in the Report of the Chief Inspector of Factories and Workshops for 1932 (Chief Inspector of Factories, 1933). By 1950, 52 cases of cancer of the nasal cavities and 93 cases of lung cancer had been reported from the refinery (Chief Inspector of Factories, 1952); these were considered by the Minister of Pensions and National Insurance to be industrial diseases. Morgan (1958) and Doll (1958) found that the relative frequency of deaths from lung cancer or cancer of the nasal cavities in these workers was significantly higher than in the male population at large. Doll et al. (1970) undertook a follow-up study of 845 men employed at the refinery for at least 5 years and who were first employed before 1944. They observed that in men employed before 1925, deaths from lung cancer were about five to ten times the numbers expected from national rates, while deaths from cancer of the nasal cavities were 100 to 900 times the expected figures. Men employed in 1925 or later showed no excess in mortality from these cancers. The results confirmed previous suggestions (Doll, 1958; Morgan, 1958) that the cancer hazard in the refinery had been effectively removed by 1925. Furthermore, among workers exposed before 1925, the risk of developing cancer of the nasal cavities persisted more or less unchanged for 15 to 42 years after the carcinogen was eliminated, whereas the risk of developing lung cancer decreased over time (Doll et al., 1970). According to data reported by the Panel on Nickel of the US National Academy of Sciences (CMBEEP, 1975), a total of 78 cases of cancer of the nasal cavities and 174 cases of lung cancer were recognized among workmen at the Clydach, Wales, nickel refinery during the 50 years from 1921 to 1971.

Twenty-four cases of cancer of the nasal cavities and 92 cases of lung cancer occurred among workmen at two nickel refineries in Ontario, Canada, during the years 1948 to 1968 (CMBEEP, 1975; Mastromatteo, 1967; Virtue, 1972). Fourteen cases of cancer of the nasal cavities, 51 cases of lung cancer and 5 cases of laryngeal cancer occurred among workmen at a nickel refinery in Kristiansand, Norway during the years 1950 to 1971 (Løken, 1950; Pedersen et al., 1973). Significant increases in the incidence of cancers of the respiratory tract have also been observed among workmen in nickel refineries in the German Democratic Republic: 45 cases of pulmonary cancers in 1932-1953 and 3 in 1972 (Konetzke, 1974a,b; Rockstroh, 1958); Japan: 19 cases of lung cancer in 1957-1959 (Tsuchiya, 1965); and the USSR (Saknyn & Shabynina, 1970, 1973; Tatarskaya, 1965, 1967; Znamenskii, 1963). Saknyn & Shabynina (1970, 1973) have also suggested that in addition to cancers of the respiratory tract, the incidence of gastric carcinomas may be higher among workers at four nickel refineries in the USSR.

The histopathologic classifications of 49 cases of lung cancer and 49 cases of nasal cavity cancer that occurred among nickel workmen have been tabulated by the Panel on Nickel of the US National Academy of Sciences (CMBEEP, 1975).

Although the exact nature of the carcinogenic agents in nickel refineries is unknown, the cancer hazard has been associated with the early stages of nickel refining which involve heavy exposure to dust from relatively crude nickel ores (Doll *et al.*, 1970). Suspicion of carcinogenicity has been focused primarily upon respirable particles of nickel subsulphide and nickel oxide and upon nickel carbonyl vapour (CMBEEP, 1975). The view that nickel carbonyl alone is responsible has been discounted due to the pronounced diminution of cancer risk despite continued use of the nickel carbonyl process after 1925 in Clydach, Wales, and due to the occurrence of excess risk of respiratory cancer among workers in nickel refineries that use the electrolytic process in lieu of the nickel carbonyl process (CMBEEP, 1975; Doll *et al.*, 1970; Mastromatteo, 1967; Pedersen *et al.*, 1973; Sunderman, 1968, 1973).

There have been three case reports of cancers of the respiratory tract in workers who were involved in nickel plating and grinding operations (Bourasset & Galland, 1966; Sunderman, 1973; Touraine & Rambaud, 1968). However, no epidemiological studies of cancer incidence have been reported among workmen who have been exposed to nickel compounds in nickel plating plants, among welders, or among workmen who have been exposed to nickel catalysts in chemical industries.

4. Comments on Data Reported and Evaluation

4.1 Animal data

Nickel subsulphide is carcinogenic in rats following its inhalation: it produced malignant lung tumours. Intramuscular injection and/or implantation of nickel subsulphide, nickel powder, nickelocene or nickel oxide, carbonate or hydroxide produced local rhabdomyosarcomas and/or fibrosarcomas in rats; nickel subsulphide and nickel oxide produced similar tumours in mice and nickel powder and nickelocene, in hamsters.

A dose-response relationship for local tumour induction after intramuscular injection of nickel subsulphide has been demonstrated in rats.

Administration of nickel carbonyl to rats by repeated intravenous injection was associated with an increased incidence of malignant tumours in various tissues. Inhalation exposure of rats to nickel carbonyl was associated with a few pulmonary malignancies.

4.2 Human data

Epidemiological studies conclusively demonstrate an excess risk of cancer of the nasal cavity and lung in workers in nickel refineries. It is likely that nickel in some form(s) is carcinogenic to man.

5. References

Adamec, J.B. & Kihlgren, T.E. (1967) Nickel and nickel alloys. In: Kirk, R.E. & Othmer, D.F., eds, Encyclopedia of Chemical Technology, 2nd ed., Vol. 13, New York, John Wiley and Sons, pp. 735-753

Antonsen, D.H. & Springer, D.B. (1967) Nickel compounds. In: Kirk, R.E. & Othmer, D.F., eds, Encyclopedia of Chemical Technology, 2nd ed., Vol. 13, New York, John Wiley and Sons, pp. 753-765

Barnett, K.W. (1974) The chemistry of nickelocene. J. organomet. Chem., 78, 139-163

Basrur, P.K. & Gilman, J.P.W. (1967) Morphologic and synthetic response of normal and tumour muscle cultures to nickel sulphide. Cancer Res., 27, 1168-1177

Beach, D.J. & Sunderman, F.W., Jr (1969) Nickel carbonyl inhibition of ^{14}C-orotic acid incorporation into rat liver RNA. Proc. Soc. exp. Biol. (N.Y.), 131, 321-322

Beach, D.J. & Sunderman, F.W., Jr (1970) Nickel carbonyl inhibition of RNA synthesis by a chromatin-RNA polymerase complex from hepatic nuclei. Cancer Res., 30, 48-50

Blaszkiewicz, G. (1967) Determination of the solubility of nickel oxide and nickel hydroxide using ^{63}Ni in water, dimethylformamide and acetonitrile. Z. Chem., 7, 245

Bourasset, A. & Galland, G. (1966) Cancer des voies respiratoires et exposition aux sels de nickel. Arch. Malad. prof., 27, 227-229

Bowen, H.J.M. (1966) Trace Elements in Biochemistry, New York, Academic Press

Broache, E.W. (1970) Nonferrous metals. In: Harper, C.A., ed., Handbook of Materials and Processes for Electronics, Section 9, New York, McGraw-Hill, pp. 59-62

Buselmaier, W. von, Röhrborn, G. & Propping, P. (1972) Mutagenitäts-Untersuchungen mit Pestiziden im Host-mediated assay und mit dem Dominanten Letaltest an der Maus. Biol. Zbl., 91, 311-325

Cajka, C.J. (1972) Nickel. In: Canadian Minerals Yearbook, Mineral Report 22, Energy, Mines and Resources, New York, International Publications Service, pp. 287-305

Chief Inspector of Factories (1933) Annual Report of the Chief Inspector of Factories for the Year 1932, London, HMSO, p.103

Chief Inspector of Factories (1952) *Annual Report of the Chief Inspector of Factories for the Year 1950*, London, HMSO, p.145

CMBEEP (Committee on Medical and Biologic Effects of Environmental Pollutants) (1975) *Nickel*, Washington DC, National Academy of Sciences

Cogley, D.R., Butler, J.N. & Synnott, J.C. (1973) Composition of non-aqueous solutions of potential use in high-energy density batteries. *AD Rep. No. 763140*, Washington DC, US National Technical Information Service

Corbett, T.H., Heidelberger, C. & Dove, W.F. (1970) Determination of the mutagenic activity to bacteriophage T4 of carcinogenic and noncarcinogenic compounds. *Mol. Pharmacol.*, 6, 667-679

Cornwall, H.R. (1966) Nickel deposits of North America. *Geological Survey Bulletin 1223*, Washington DC, US Government Printing Office, pp. 1-62

Cornwall, H.R. (1973) *Nickel*. In: Brobst, D.A. & Pratt, W.P., eds, *United States Mineral Resources*, Geological Survey Professional Paper 820, Washington DC, US Government Printing Office, pp.437-442

Corrick, J.D. (1973) *Nickel*. Preprint from the *1973 Bureau of Mines Minerals Yearbook*, Washington DC, US Department of the Interior, pp. 1-15

Daniel, M.R. (1966) Strain differences in the response of rats to the injection of nickel sulphide. *Brit. J. Cancer*, 20, 886-895

Dean, J.G. (1959) The industrial growth of nickel compounds. *Industr. Eng. Chem.*, 51, 48A-53A

Doll, R. (1958) Cancer of the lung and nose in nickel workers. *Brit. J. industr. Med.*, 15, 217-223

Doll, R., Morgan, L.G. & Speizer, F.E. (1970) Cancers of the lung and nasal sinuses in nickel workers. *Brit. J. Cancer*, 24, 623-632

Eméleus, H.J. (1950) *Nonvolatile inorganic fluorides*. In: Simons, J.H., ed., *Fluorine Chemistry*, Vol. 1, New York, Academic Press, pp.63-69

Fairbridge, R.W., ed. (1974) *The Encyclopedia of Geochemistry and Environmental Sciences*, Vol. IVA, New York, Van Nostrand-Reinhold, pp.790-793

Falk, H.L. (1970) *Chemical definitions of inhalation hazards*. In: Hanna, M.G., Jr, Nettesheim, P. & Gilbert, J.R., eds, *Inhalation Carcinogenesis*, US Atomic Energy Commission Symposium Series No. 18, Oak Ridge, Tenn., US AEC Division of Technical Information Extension, pp.13-26

Farrell, R.L. & Davis, G.W. (1974) *The effects of particulates on respiratory carcinogenesis by diethylnitrosamine*. In: Karbe, E. & Park, J.F., eds, *Experimental Lung Cancer: Carcinogenesis and Bioassays*, New York, Springer-Verlag, pp.219-233

Fischer, A. (1967) Preparation of metal sulfamates. US Patent 3,321,273, Tenneco Chemicals Inc.

Furst, A. & Schlauder, M.C. (1971) The hamster as a model for metal carcinogenesis. Proc. West. Pharmacol. Soc., 14, 68-71

Furst, A., Cassetta, D.M. & Sasmore, D.P. (1973) Rapid induction of pleural mesotheliomas in the rat. Proc. West. Pharmacol. Soc., 16, 150-153

Gilman, J.P.W. (1962) Metal carcinogenesis. II. A study of the carcinogenic activity of cobalt, copper, iron and nickel compounds. Cancer Res., 22, 158-162

Gilman, J.P.W. (1966) Muscle tumourigenesis. Canad. Cancer Conf., 6, 209-223

Gilman, J.P.W. & Herchen, H. (1963) The effect of physical form of implant on nickel sulphide tumourigenesis in the rat. Un. int. cancr. acta, 19, 615-619

Gilman, J.P.W. & Ruckerbauer, G.M. (1962) Metal carcinogenesis. I. Observations on the carcinogenicity of a refinery dust, cobalt oxide and colloidal thorium dioxide. Cancer Res., 22, 152-157

Hackett, R.L. & Sunderman, F.W., Jr (1969) Nickel carbonyl. Effects upon the ultrastructure of hepatic parenchymal cells. Arch. environm. Hlth, 19, 337-343

Haendler, H.M., Patterson, W.L., Jr & Bernard, W.J. (1952) The reaction of fluorine with zinc, nickel and some of their binary compounds. Some properties of zinc and nickel fluorides. J. Amer. chem. Soc., 74, 3167-3168

Heath, J.C. & Daniel, M.R. (1964) The production of malignant tumours by nickel in the rat. Brit. J. Cancer, 18, 261-264

Herchen, H. & Gilman, J.P.W. (1964) Effect of duration of exposure on nickel sulphide tumourigenesis. Nature (Lond.), 202, 306-307

Hueper, W.C. (1952) Experimental studies in metal carcinogenesis. I. Nickel cancers in rats. Texas Rep. Biol. Med., 10, 167-186

Hueper, W.C. (1955) Experimental studies in metal carcinogenesis. IV. Cancer produced by parenterally introduced metallic nickel. J. nat. Cancer Inst., 16, 55-73

Hueper, W.C. (1958) Experimental studies in metal carcinogenesis. IX. Pulmonary lesions in guinea pigs and rats exposed to prolonged inhalation of powdered metallic nickel. Arch. Path., 65, 600-607

Hueper, W.C. & Payne, W.W. (1962) Experimental studies in metal carcinogenesis: chromium, nickel, iron and arsenic. Arch. environm. Hlth, 5, 445-462

IARC (1973) IARC Monographs on the Evaluation of Carcinogenic Risk of Chemicals to Man, Vol. 2, Some inorganic and organometallic compounds, Lyon, pp.126-149

Jasmin, G. (1963) Effects of methandrostenolone on muscle carcinogenesis induced in rats by nickel sulphide. Brit. J. Cancer, 17, 681-686

Jasmin, G. (1965) Influence of age, sex and glandular extirpation on muscle carcinogenesis in rats. Experientia, 21, 149-150

Jasmin, G., Bajusz, E. & Mongeau, A. (1963) Influence du sexe et de la castration sur la production de tumeurs musculaires chez le rat par le sulfure de nickel. Rev. Canad. Biol., 22, 113-114

Kasprzak, K.S., Marchow, L. & Breborowicz, J. (1973) Pathological reactions in rat lungs following intratracheal injection of nickel subsulphide and 3,4-benzpyrene. Res. Commun. chem. Path. Pharmacol., 6, 237-245

Knox, G.R., Munro, J.D., Paulson, P.L., Smith, G.H. & Watts, W.E. (1961) Some substituted cyclopentadienyl derivatives of nickel, cobalt, iron, molybdenum and titanium. J. chem. Soc., 4619-4624

Konetzke, G.W. (1974a) Berufliche Krebserkrankungen durch Arsen und Nickel sowei deren Verbindungen. Dtsch. Ges. Wesen, 29, 1334

Konetzke, G.W. (1974b) Die kanzerogene Wirkung von Arsen und Nickel. Arch. Geschwulstforsch., 44, 16-22

Lau, T.J., Hackett, R.L. & Sunderman, F.W., Jr (1972) The carcinogenicity of intravenous nickel carbonyl in rats. Cancer Res., 32, 2253-2258

Lewis, C.L. & Ott, W.L. (1970) Analytical chemistry of nickel, International Series of Monographs in Analytical Chemistry, Vol. 43, New York, Pergamon

Løken, A.C. (1950) Lung cancer in nickel workers. Tidsskr. Norske Laegefor., 70, 376-378

Maenza, R.M., Pradham, A.M. & Sunderman, F.W., Jr (1971) Rapid induction of sarcomas in rats by a combination of nickel sulphide and 3,4-benzpyrene. Cancer Res., 31, 2067-2071

Mason, M.M. (1972) Nickel sulphide carcinogenesis. Environm. Physiol. Biochem., 2, 137-141

Mason, M.M., Cate, C.C. & Baker, J. (1971) Toxicology and carcinogenesis of various chemicals used in the preparation of vaccines. Clin. Toxicol., 4, 185-204

Mastromatteo, E. (1967) Nickel: a review of its occupational health aspects. J. occup. Med., 9, 127-136

McMurdie, H.F., Morris, M.C., deGroot, J. & Swanson, H.E. (1971) Crystallography of some double sulfates and chromates. J. Res. nat. US Bur. Standards, 75A, 435-439

Mitchell, D.F., Shankwalker, G.B. & Shazer, S. (1960) Determining the tumourigenicity of dental materials. J. dent. Res., 39, 1023-1028

Morgan, J.G. (1958) Some observations on the incidence of respiratory cancer in nickel workers. Brit. J. industr. Med., 15, 224-234

Natusch, D.F.S., Wallace, J.R. & Evans, C.A., Jr (1974) Toxic trace elements: preferential concentration in respirable particles. Science, 183, 202-204

Olinici, C.D., Risca, R. & Todorutiu, C. (1973) Observatii citogenetice asupra tumorilor induse cu nichel la sobolani. Oncol. radiolog., 12, 41-46

Ottolenghi, A.D., Haseman, J.K., Payne, W.W., Falk, H.L. & MacFarland, H.N. (1975) Inhalation studies of nickel sulfide in pulmonary carcinogenesis of rats. J. nat. Cancer Inst., 54, 1165-1172

Paulson, P.L. (1955) Ferrocene and related compounds. Quart. Revs, 9, 391-403

Payne, W.W. (1964) Carcinogenicity of nickel compounds in experimental animals. Proc. Amer. Ass. Cancer Res., 5, 50

Pedersen, E., Høgetveit, A.C. & Andersen, A. (1973) Cancer of respiratory organs among workers at a nickel refinery in Norway. Int. J. Cancer, 12, 32-41

Peshkova, V.M. & Savostina, V.N. (1971) Analytical Chemistry of Nickel, New York, Halsted

Rockstroh, H. von (1958) Zur Aetiologie des Bronchialkrebses in arsenverarbeitenden Nickelhütten. Arch. Geschwulstforsch., 14, 151-162

Sachdev, S.L. & West, P.W. (1970) Concentration of trace metals by solvent extraction and their determination by atomic absorption spectrophotometry. Environm. Sci. Technol., 4, 749-751

Saknyn, A.V. & Shabynina, N.K. (1970) Some statistical data on carcinogenous hazards for workers engaged in the production of nickel from oxidized ores. Gig. Trud. Prof. Zabol., 14, 10-13

Saknyn, A.V. & Shabynina, N.K. (1973) Epidemiology of malignant neoplasms at nickel smelters. Gig. Trud. Prof. Zabol., 17, 25-29

Sandell, E.B. (1959) Colorimetric Determination of Traces of Metals, 3rd ed., New York, Interscience, pp. 665-681

Santmyers, D. & Aarons, R. (1967) Sulfamic acid and sulfamates. In: Kirk, R.E. & Othmer, D.F., eds, Encyclopedia of Chemical Technology, 2nd ed., Vol. 19, New York, John Wiley and Sons, pp.242-249

Schroeder, H.A. (1970) Nickel. Air Quality Monograph #70-14, Washington DC, American Petroleum Institute, pp.1-24

Schroeder, H.A., Balassa, J.J. & Tipton, I.H. (1961) Abnormal trace metals in man: nickel. J. chron. Dis., 15, 51-65

Stacey, M., Tatlow, J.C. & Sharpe, A.G., eds (1960) Advances in Fluorine Chemistry, Vol. 1, London, Butterworths Scientific Publications, pp.84-88

Stecher, P., ed. (1968) The Merck Index, 8th ed., Rahway, NJ, Merck & Co., pp.727-728

Stephen, H. & Stephen, T., eds (1963) Solubilities of Inorganic and Organic Compounds, Vol. 1, parts 1 and 2, New York, Macmillan, pp. 52-53, 228, 355-358, 1010-1012

Sullivan, R.J. (1969) Air Pollution Aspects of Nickel and its Compounds, Technical Report, Bethesda, Litton Systems Inc.

Sunderman, F.W. & Donnelly, A.J. (1965) Studies of nickel carcinogenesis. Metastasizing pulmonary tumors in rats induced by the inhalation of nickel carbonyl. Amer. J. clin. Path., 46, 1027-1041

Sunderman, F.W. & Sunderman, F.W., Jr (1961) Nickel poisoning. XI. Implication of nickel as a pulmonary carcinogen in tobacco smoke. Amer. J. clin. Path., 35, 203-209

Sunderman, F.W., Kincaid, J.F., Donnelly, A.J. & West, B. (1957) Nickel poisoning. IV. Chronic exposure of rats to nickel carbonyl: a report after one year of observation. Arch. industr. Hlth, 16, 480-485

Sunderman, F.W., Donnelly, A.J., West, B. & Kincaid, J.F. (1959) Nickel poisoning. IX. Carcinogenesis in rats exposed to nickel carbonyl. Arch. industr. Hlth, 20, 36-41

Sunderman, F.W., Jr (1963) Studies of nickel carcinogenesis: alterations of ribonucleic acid following inhalation of nickel carbonyl. Amer. J. clin. Path., 39, 549-561

Sunderman, F.W., Jr (1967a) Nickel carbonyl inhibition of cortisone induction of hepatic tryptophan pyrrolase. Cancer Res., 27, 1595-1599

Sunderman, F.W., Jr (1967b) Inhibition of induction of benzpyrene hydroxylase by nickel carbonyl. Cancer Res., 27, 950-955

Sunderman, F.W., Jr (1968) Nickel carcinogenesis. Epidemiology of respiratory cancer among nickel workers. Dis. Chest, 54, 41

Sunderman, F.W., Jr (1971) Metal carcinogenesis in experimental animals. Fd Cosmet. Toxicol., 9, 105-120

Sunderman, F.W., Jr (1973) The current status of nickel carcinogenesis. Ann. clin. Lab. Sci., 3, 156-180

Sunderman, F.W., Jr (1976) Metal carcinogenesis. In: Goyer, R.A. & Mehlman, M.A., eds, Advances in Modern Toxicology, Washington DC, Hemisphere Publishing Corp. (in press)

Sunderman, F.W., Jr & Maenza, R.M. (1976) Comparisons of the carcinogenicities of nickel subsulphide (Ni_3S_2), nickel sulphide (NiS), nickel dust, iron dust, and nickel-iron sulphide (NiFeS) following i.m. administration in Fischer rats. Proc. Amer. Ass. Cancer Res. (in press)

Sunderman, F.W., Jr & Sunderman, F.W. (1963) Studies of pulmonary carcinogenesis: the sub-cellular partition of nickel and the binding of ribonucleic acid. Fed. Proc., 22, 427

Sunderman, F.W., Jr, Roszel, N.O. & Clark, R.J. (1968) Gas chromatography of nickel carbonyl in blood and breath. Arch. environm. Hlth, 16, 836-843

Sunderman, F.W., Jr, Lau, T.J. & Cralley, L.J. (1974) Inhibitory effect of manganese upon muscle tumorigenesis by nickel subsulphide. Cancer Res., 34, 92-95

Sunderman, F.W., Jr, Lau, T.J., Minghetti, P.F., Maenza, R.M., Becker, N., Onkelinx, C. & Goldblatt, P.J. (1975) Effects of manganese on tumorigenesis and metabolism of nickel subsulphide. Proc. Amer. Ass. Cancer Res., 16, 554

Sunderman, F.W., Jr, Kasprzak, K.S., Lau, T.J., Minghetti, P.F., Maenza, R.M., Becker, N., Onkelinx, C. & Goldblatt, P.J. (1976) Effects of manganese on carcinogenicity and metabolism of nickel subsulphide. Cancer Res. (in press)

Swierenga, S.H.H. (1970) The role of nickel in the induction of muscle tumours (Doctoral Dissertation, University of Guelph, Ontario)

Swierenga, S.H.H. & Basrur, P.K. (1968) Effect of nickel on cultured rat embryo muscle cells. Lab. Invest., 19, 663-674

Szadkowski, D., Schultze, H., Schaller, K.H. & Lehnert, G. (1969) Zur ökologischen Bedeutung des Schwermetallgehaltes von Zigaretten. Blei-, Cadmium- und Nickelanalysen des Tabaks sowie der Gas- und Partikelphase. Arch. Hyg. (München), 153, 1-8

Tatarskaya, A.A. (1965) Occupational cancer of upper respiratory passages in the nickel industry. Gig. Trud. Prof. Zabol., 9, 22-25

Tatarskaya, A.A. (1967) Cancer of the respiratory tract in people engaged in nickel industry. Vop. Onkol., 13, 58-60

Touraine, R. & Rambaud, G. (1968) Les cancers bronchiques primitifs à localisation double unilatérale. J. fr. Med. Chirurg. thorac., 22, 757-767

Tsuchiya, K. (1965) The relation of occupation to cancer, especially cancer of the lung. Cancer, 18, 136-144

US Bureau of Mines (1975) Minerals in the US Economy, General Publication 1975:3,C2, Washington DC, US Department of the Interior

US Department of Commerce (1974) US Imports for Consumption and General Imports, FT 246/Annual 1973, Washington DC, US Government Printing Office, p.344

Virtue, J.A. (1972) The relationship between the refining of nickel and cancer of the nasal cavity. Canad. J. Otolaryng., 1, 37-42

Watanabe, H., Motoyama, I. & Hata, K. (1965) Simple method for preparing metallocenes. Bull. chem. Soc. Japan, 38, 853-854

Weast, R.C., ed. (1975) Handbook of Chemistry and Physics, 56th ed., Cleveland, Ohio, The Chemical Rubber Company

Webb, M. & Weinzierl, S.M. (1972) Uptake of $^{63}Ni^{2+}$ from its complexes with proteins and other ligands by mouse dermal fibroblasts *in vitro*. Brit. J. Cancer, 26, 292-298

Webb, M., Heath, J.C. & Hopkins, T. (1972) Intramuscular distribution of the inducing metal in primary rhabdomyosarcomata induced in the rat by nickel, cobalt and cadmium. Brit. J. Cancer, 26, 274-278

Wehner, A.P. (1974) Investigation of Cocarcinogenicity of Asbestos, Cobalt Oxide, Nickel Oxide, Diethylnitrosamine and Cigarette Smoke (Final Report to the National Cancer Institute on Contract PH 43-68-1372), Richland, Washington, Battelle Pacific Northwest Laboratories

Wehner, A.P., Busch, R.H., Olson, R.J. & Craig, D.K. (1975) Chronic inhalation of nickel oxide and cigarette smoke by hamsters. Amer. industr. Hyg. Ass. J., 36, 801-810

Weinzierl, S.M. & Webb, M. (1972) Interaction of carcinogenic metals with tissue and body fluids. Brit. J. Cancer, 26, 279-291

Witschi, H. (1972) A comparative study of *in vivo* RNA and protein synthesis in rat liver and lung. Cancer Res., 32, 1686-1694

Znamenskii, S.V. (1963) Occupational bronchogenic cancers in workers extracting, isolating and reprocessing nickel ore. Vop. Onkol., 9, 130

EPOXIDES

DIEPOXYBUTANE*

1. Chemical and Physical Data

1.1 Synonyms and trade names

(a) Diepoxybutane

Chem. Abstr. Reg. Serial No.: 1464-53-5

Chem. Abstr. Name: 2,2'-Bioxirane

1,1'-Bi(ethylene oxide); butadiene diepoxide; butadiene dioxide; 2,4-diepoxybutane; 1,2:3,4-diepoxybutane; dioxybutadiene; erythritol anhydride

Bioxiran; Bioxirane

(b) DL-1,2:3,4-Diepoxybutane

Chem. Abstr. Reg. Serial No.: 298-18-0

Chem. Abstr. Name: (R*,R*)-(+-)-2,2'-Bioxirane

1,2:3,4-Dianhydro-DL-threitol; (+-)-1,2:3,4-diepoxybutane; DL-1,2:3,4-diepoxybutane; D,L-diepoxybutane

(c) D-1,2:3,4-Diepoxybutane

Chem. Abstr. Reg. Serial No.: 30419-67-1

Chem. Abstr. Name: [R-(R*,R*)]-2,2'-Bioxirane

1,2:3,4-Dianhydro-D-threitol; D-diepoxybutane; (2R,3R)-diepoxybutane; (2R,3R)-1,2:3,4-diepoxybutane

(d) L-1,2:3,4-Diepoxybutane

Chem. Abstr. Reg. Serial No.: 30031-64-2

Chem. Abstr. Name: [S-(R*,R*)]-2,2'-Bioxirane

1,2:3,4-Dianhydro-L-threitol; (2S,3S)-diepoxybutane; L-diepoxybutane; (2S,3S)-1,2:3,4-diepoxybutane

---

*Considered by the Working Group, February 1976

(e) *meso*-1,2:3,4-Diepoxybutane

Chem. Abstr. Reg. Serial No.: 564-00-1

Chem. Abstr. Name: (R*,S*)-2,2'-Bioxirane

1,2:3,4-Dianhydroerythritol; *meso*-diepoxybutane; (R*,S*)-diepoxybutane

1.2 Chemical formula and molecular weight

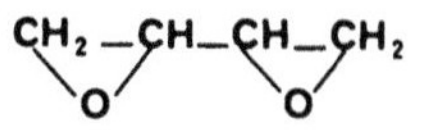

$$CH_2-CH-CH-CH_2$$
$$\diagdown O \diagup \quad \diagdown O \diagup$$

$C_4H_6O_2$ Mol. wt: 86.1

1.3 Chemical and physical properties

(a) Description: Colourless liquid

(b) Boiling-point: 138°C; 140-142°C (*meso*-form)

(c) Melting-point: 4°C (DL-form); 19°C (*meso*-form)

(d) Density: d_4^{18} 1.113

(e) Refractive index: n_D^{20} 1.4289 (DL-form); n_D^{23} 1.4272 (*meso*-form) (Van Duuren *et al.*, 1963)

(f) Spectroscopy data: Infra-red epoxide band at 1250 cm^{-1}

(g) Solubility: Miscible with water

(h) Stability: Slowly hydrolysed in water to erythritol or threitol

(i) Reactivity: Reacts with 4-(4'-nitrobenzyl)pyridine (Preussmann *et al.*, 1969)

1.4 Technical products and impurities

No data were available to the Working Group.

2. Production, Use, Occurrence and Analysis

For important background information on this section, see preamble, p. 19.

2.1 Production and use

Diepoxybutane was prepared in 1884 by treatment of erythrityl chlorohydrin with alkali. It has since been made by reacting 1,4-dichloro-2,3-butanediol or a 2,3-dihalogeno-1,4-butanediol with sodium hydroxide. The DL-form has been prepared from 1,4-dibromo-2-butene and the *meso*-form from 1,4-dihydroxy-2-butene or 3,4-epoxy-1-butene (Shostakovskii *et al.*, 1966; Stecher, 1968). The L-form has been prepared from (2S,3S)-threitol 1,4-bis-methanesulphonate *via* (2S,3S)-1,2-epoxy-3,4-butanediol 4-methanesulphonate (Feit *et al.*, 1970).

In some countries diepoxybutane has been used in the curing of polymers, for cross-linking textile fibres and in the prevention of microbial spoilage (Stecher, 1968). Several patents have been issued on its use in polymer, paper and textile treatments and as a chemical intermediate.

2.2 Occurrence

No data were available to the Working Group.

2.3 Analysis

See section 'General Remarks on the Substances Considered', p. 29.

3. Biological Data Relevant to the Evaluation of Carcinogenic Risk to Man

3.1 Carcinogenicity and related studies in animals

(a) Skin application

Mouse: Two groups of 30 8-week old male ICR/Ha Swiss mice were given thrice weekly skin applications on the clipped dorsal skin of 10 mg/animal D,L- or *meso*-1,2:3,4-diepoxybutane in 0.1 ml acetone. Median survival times were 78 and 154 days, respectively. With D,L-diepoxybutane, 2 mice developed skin tumours; one of these had a squamous-cell carcinoma. With the *meso* isomer, 6 mice developed skin tumours; 4 of these had squamous-cell carcinomas. Among 90 solvent control mice 8 developed skin papillomas (Van Duuren *et al.*, 1963).

In another experiment, two groups of 30 8-week old female ICR/Ha Swiss mice received 3 and 10 mg of D,L-1,2:3,4-diepoxybutane in 0.1 ml acetone, respectively, applied on the clipped dorsal skin thrice weekly for lifespan. One mouse given the higher dose developed a skin papilloma (mean survival time, 165 days). Of mice given the lower dose, 10 developed skin papillomas and 6 developed squamous-cell carcinomas of the skin (mean survival time, 475 days). *meso*-1,2:3,4-Diepoxybutane was tested at the same doses: 5 animals at the higher dose developed skin papillomas and 4 developed squamous-cell carcinomas of the skin. At the lower dose 1 animal developed a skin papilloma; there were no carcinomas. No skin tumours occurred in 60 acetone-treated controls (Van Duuren *et al.*, 1965).

(b) Subcutaneous and/or intramuscular administration

Mouse: In groups of 50 and 30 8-week old female ICR/Ha Swiss mice given s.c. injections of 0.1 or 1.1 mg/animal D,L-1,2:3,4-diepoxybutane in tricaprylin once weekly for over a year, 5/50 and 5/30 mice, respectively, developed local fibrosarcomas. The mean survival times were 456 and 328 days. No local sarcomas developed in 3 groups of solvent-treated controls (Van Duuren *et al.*, 1966).

Rat: Of 50 6-week old female Sprague-Dawley rats given once weekly s.c. injections of 1 mg D,L-1,2:3,4-diepoxybutane in tricaprylin, 9 animals developed local fibrosarcomas; the median survival time was 470 days. No local tumours developed in 50 solvent-injected controls (Van Duuren *et al.*, 1966).

(c) Intraperitoneal administration

Mouse: Groups of 15 male and 15 female 4-6-week old A/J mice were given 12 thrice weekly i.p. injections of L-1,2:3,4-diepoxybutane dissolved in water or in tricaprylin. Total doses in water were 1.7, 6.7, 27, 108 and 192 mg/kg bw, and the resulting incidences of lung tumours were 21, 40, 55, 64 and 78%, respectively (0.2, 0.5, 0.8, 0.9 and 1.5 tumours per mouse). Total doses in tricaprylin were 3, 12, 48 and 192 mg/kg bw, and the resulting incidences of lung tumours were 40, 43, 46 and 50%, respectively (0.5, 0.6, 0.8 and 0.75 tumours per mouse). Of 447 controls injected with water or tricaprylin, 35% had lung tumours, with 0.44 tumours per mouse

(Shimkin et al., 1966) [The increases in numbers of lung tumours were significant (P<0.01) at the 3 highest dose levels administered in water].

3.2 Other relevant biological data

(a) Experimental systems

(i) Diepoxybutane (mixed steroisomers): The oral LD_{50} in rats is 78 mg/kg bw (Smyth et al., 1954) and the percutaneous LD_{50} in rabbits is 98 mg/kg bw. In rats, the LC_{50} is 371 mg/m^3 (90 ppm) for a 4-hour exposure. Exposure caused lachrymation, clouding of the cornea, laboured breathing and congestion of the lungs. Surviving animals gained weight less rapidly than controls during recovery and suffered from atrophy of the thymus and involution of the spleen (Hine & Rowe, 1963).

In mice, toxicity and a high rate of mortality have been associated with percutaneous tests involving application of an acetone or arachis oil solution of 1,2:3,4-diepoxybutane (Hendry et al., 1951). In rabbits, diepoxybutane is an eye irritant, produces burns and blisters on the skin and causes extreme irritation of the pulmonary tract. Six intramuscular injections of 25 mg/kg bw produced leucopenia and lymphopenia (Hine & Rowe, 1963).

Diepoxybutane alkylates DNA primarily at the N-7 position of guanine (Van Duuren, 1969).

It produced 97% inhibition of the growth of Walker carcinoma in rats (Hendry et al., 1951).

Diepoxybutane induced prophage in *Bacillus megaterium* and *Pseudomonas pyocyanea* (Lwoff, 1953) and in *Escherichia coli* k-12 (Heinemann & Howard, 1964). It induced reverse mutations in strain TA 1535 of *Salmonella typhimurium* (McCann et al., 1975), in *Schizosaccharomyces pombe* (Clarke & Loprieno, 1965) and in B and B/r strains of *Escherichia coli* after treatment for 1 hour at 37°C with 0.01 M and 0.02 M aqueous solutions, respectively (Glover, 1956). Reverse mutations were also induced in the purple, adenine-requiring mutant 38701 of *Neurospora crassa* after treatment with a 0.2 M solution (Kølmark & Westergaard, 1953).

The compound produced mitotic gene conversions in strain D4 of *Saccharomyces cerevisiae* after 5 hours of treatment with a 0.005 M solution (Zimmermann, 1971; Zimmermann & Vig, 1975). In *Drosophila melanogaster* it has produced sex-linked recessive lethal mutations, visible mutations, semi-lethal mutations (Bird & Fahmy, 1953), translocations (Watson, 1966, 1972) and minute mutations (Fahmy & Fahmy, 1970).

Diepoxybutane produced chromosome aberrations in cells taken from a patient suffering from Fanconi's anaemia which were treated *in vitro* for 7 days (Wolman & Auerbach, 1975).

(ii) D,L-1,2:3,4-Diepoxybutane: In rats, a solution of 5 mg D,L-1,2:3,4-diepoxybutane in 0.5 ml tricaprylin administered intragastrically once weekly for a year was non-toxic (Van Duuren et al., 1966); in mice, skin damage was seen (Van Duuren et al., 1963).

(iii) L-1,2:3,4-Diepoxybutane: The i.p. LD_{50} in strain A/J mice is 16 mg/kg bw (Shimkin et al., 1966).

(iv) *meso*-1,2:3,4-Diepoxybutane: The i.p. LD_{50} in mice is 25 mg/kg bw (Stecher, 1968). It produces 55% inhibition of the growth of Walker carcinoma in rats (Hendry et al., 1951).

The mutagenicity of the individual steroisomers of diepoxybutane has been tested only in plants, in which they have been found to be mutagenic (Bianchi & Contin, 1962; Ehrenberg & Gustafsson, 1957).

(b) Man

In man, minor, accidental exposure to diepoxybutane (mixed stereo-isomers) caused swelling of the eyelids, painful eye irritation and upper respiratory tract irritation within 6 hours (Hine & Rowe, 1963).

3.3 Observations in man

No data were available to the Working Group.

4. Comments on Data Reported and Evaluation[1]

4.1 Animal data

D,L- and *meso*-1,2:3,4-diepoxybutane are carcinogenic in mice by skin application: both compounds produced squamous-cell skin carcinomas. The D,L-racemate also produced local sarcomas in mice and rats by subcutaneous injection. L-1,2:3,4-Diepoxybutane is carcinogenic in mice by intraperitoneal injection.

4.2 Human data

No case reports or epidemiological studies were available to the Working Group.

---

[1]See also the section 'Animal Data in Relation to the Evaluation of Risk to Man' in the introduction to this volume, p. 17.

5. References

Bianchi, A. & Contin, M. (1962) Mutagenic activity of isomeric forms of diepoxybutane in maize. J. Heredity, 53, 277-281

Bird, M.J. & Fahmy, O.G. (1953) Cytogenetic analysis of the action of carcinogens and tumour inhibitors in *Drosophila melanogaster*. I. 1:2,3:4-Diepoxybutane. Proc. roy. Soc., Ser. B, 140B, 556-578

Clarke, C.H. & Loprieno, N. (1965) The influence of genetic background on the induction of methionine reversions by diepoxybutane in *Schizosaccharomyces pombe*. Microb. Genet. Bull., 22, 11-12

Ehrenberg, L. & Gustafsson, A. (1957) On the mutagenic action of ethylene oxide and diepoxybutane in barley. Hereditas, 43, 595-602

Fahmy, O.G. & Fahmy, M.J. (1970) Gene elimination in carcinogenesis: reinterpretation of the somatic mutation theory. Cancer Res., 30, 195-205

Feit, P.W., Rastrup-Andersen, N. & Matagne, R. (1970) Epoxide formation from (2S,3S)-threitol 1,4-bis-methanesulfonate. J. med. Chem., 13, 1173-1175

Glover, S.W. (1956) A comparative study of induced reversions in *Escherichia coli*. In: Genetic Studies with Bacteria, Carnegie Institution of Washington Publication 612, Washington DC, pp. 121-136

Heinemann, B. & Howard, A.J. (1964) Induction of lambda-bacteriophage in *Escherichia coli* as a screening test for potential antitumor agents. Appl. Microbiol., 12, 234-239

Hendry, J.A., Homer, R.F., Rose, F.L. & Walpole, A.L. (1951) Cytotoxic agents. II. Bis-epoxides and related compounds. Brit. J. Pharmacol., 6, 235-255

Hine, C.H. & Rowe, V.K. (1963) Butadiene dioxide. In: Patty, F.A., ed., Industrial Hygiene and Toxicology, 2nd ed., Vol. 2, New York, Interscience pp. 1600-1601

Kølmark, G. & Westergaard, M. (1953) Further studies on chemically induced reversions at the adenine locus of *Neurospora*. Hereditas, 39, 209-224

Lwoff, A. (1953) Lysogeny. Bact. Rev., 17, 269-337

McCann, J., Choi, E., Yamasaki, E. & Ames, B.N. (1975) Detection of carcinogens as mutagens in the *Salmonella*/microsome test: assay of 300 chemicals Proc. nat. Acad. Sci. (Wash.), 72, 5135-5139

Preussmann, R., Schneider, H. & Epple, F. (1969) Untersuchungen zum Nachweis alkylierender Agentien. II. Der Nachweis verschiedener Klassen alkylierender Agentien mit einer Modifikation der Farbreaktion mit 4-(4'-Nitrobenzyl)pyridin (NBP). Arzneimittelforsch., 19, 1059-1073

Shimkin, M.B., Weisburger, J.H., Weisburger, E.K., Gubareff, N. & Suntzeff, V. (1966) Bioassay of 29 alkylating chemicals by the pulmonary-tumor response in strain A mice. J. nat. Cancer Inst., 36, 915-935

Shostakovskii, M.F., Atavin, A.S., Trofimov, B.A. & Nikitin, V.M. (1966) Butadiene dioxide. USSR Patent 185,873, September 12

Smyth, H.F., Jr, Carpenter, C.P., Weil, C.S. & Pozzani, U.C. (1954) Range-finding toxicity data. Arch. industr. Hyg., 10, 61-68

Stecher, P.G., ed. (1968) The Merck Index, 8th ed., Rahway, NJ, Merck & Co., p. 418

Van Duuren, B.L. (1969) Carcinogenic epoxides, lactones and halo-ethers and their mode of action. Ann. N.Y. Acad. Sci., 163, 633-651

Van Duuren, B.L., Nelson, N., Orris, L., Palmes, E.D. & Schmitt, F.L. (1963) Carcinogenicity of epoxides, lactones and peroxy compounds. J. nat. Cancer Inst., 31, 41-55

Van Duuren, B.L., Orris, L. & Nelson, N. (1965) Carcinogenicity of epoxides, lactones and peroxy compounds. II. J. nat. Cancer Inst., 35, 707-717

Van Duuren, B.L., Langseth, L., Orris, L., Teebor, G., Nelson, N. & Kuschner, M. (1966) Carcinogenicity of epoxides, lactones and peroxy compounds. IV. Tumor response in epithelial and connective tissue in mice and rats. J. nat. Cancer Inst., 37, 825-838

Watson, W.A.F. (1966) Further evidence of an essential difference between the genetical effects of mono- and bifunctional alkylating agents. Mutation Res., 3, 455-457

Watson, W.A.F. (1972) Studies on a recombination-deficient mutation of Drosophila. II. Response to X-rays and alkylating agents. Mutation Res., 14, 299-307

Wolman, S.R. & Auerbach, A.D. (1975) Induction of chromosome damage in fibroblasts from genetic instability syndromes. Proc. Amer. Ass. Cancer Res., 16, 69

Zimmermann, F.K. (1971) Induction of mitotic gene conversion by mutagens. Mutation Res., 11, 327-337

Zimmermann, F.K. & Vig, B.K. (1975) Mutagen specificity in the induction of mitotic crossing over in Saccharomyces cerevisiae. Mol. gen. Genet., 139, 255-268

DIGLYCIDYL RESORCINOL ETHER*

1. Chemical and Physical Data

1.1 Synonyms and trade names

Chem. Abstr. Reg. Serial No.: 101-90-6

Chem. Abstr. Name: 2,2'-[1,3-Phenylene bis(oxymethylene)]bis-oxirane

1,3-Bis(2,3-epoxypropoxy)benzene; *meta*-bis(2,3-epoxypropoxy)-benzene; RDGE: resorcinol diglycidyl ether; resorcinyl diglycidyl ether

Araldite ERE 1359

1.2 Chemical formula and molecular weight

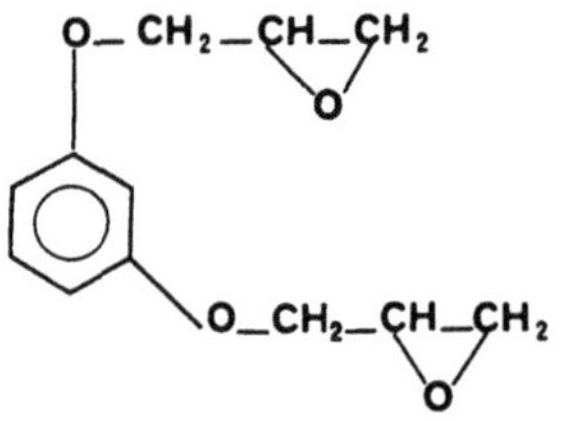

$C_{12}H_{14}O_4$ Mol. wt: 222.2

1.3 Chemical and physical properties

From Hawley (1971)

(a) Description: Pale-yellow liquid
(b) Boiling-point: 172°C at 0.8 mm
(c) Density: d_4^{25} 1.21
(d) Refractive index: n_D^{25} 1.541

---

*Considered by the Working Group, February 1976

1.4 Technical products and impurities

Typical properties of commercial diglycidyl resorcinol ether are a viscosity of 300-500 centipoises (25°C) and an epoxy equivalent of 130. Specifications for commercial diglycidyl resorcinol ether in Japan are a minimum of 98.5% non-volatile matter, and an epoxy equivalent of 125-135.

2. Production, Use, Occurrence and Analysis

For important background information on this section, see preamble, p. 19.

2.1 Production and use

Diglycidyl resorcinol ether was synthesized in 1948 by the reaction of an excess of epichlorohydrin with resorcinol in alkaline solution (Werner & Farenhorst, 1948), and this is believed to be the method used for commercial production.

Although there are two producers of this chemical in the US, the quantity produced is not known; one company started production in 1974. One company in Japan started producing this compound in 1974, and an estimated 5 thousand kg were produced in 1975.

Diglycidyl resorcinol ether is used as a liquid epoxy resin and as a reactive diluent in the production of other epoxy resins (Lee & Neville, 1967). Cured resins made from it have been reported to have characteristics which make them useful for electrical, casting, tooling, adhesive and laminating applications and as a coating for metal and certain pavements to increase tensile strength. It has also been used to cure polysulphide rubber.

2.2 Occurrence

No data were available to the Working Group.

2.3 Analysis

See section 'General Remarks on the Substances Considered', p. 29.

3. Biological Data Relevant to the Evaluation of Carcinogenic Risk to Man

3.1 Carcinogenicity and related studies in animals

(a) *Skin application*

Mouse: In a preliminary report, McCammon et al. (1957) stated that a significant number of skin tumours were produced in C57Bl mice by thrice weekly skin painting of diglycidyl resorcinol ether [The study was not fully reported and cannot be evaluated].

No skin tumours occurred in 30 8-week old female Swiss ICR/Ha mice which received thrice weekly skin paintings of a 1% solution in benzene (approximately 0.1 ml solution per application) for life; the median survival time was 491 days (Van Duuren et al., 1965).

(b) *Subcutaneous and/or intramuscular administration*

Rat: In a preliminary report McCammon et al. (1957) reported that s.c. injection of diglycidyl resorcinol ether resulted in a statistically significant increase in the numbers of local tumours in Long-Evans rats [The study was not fully reported and cannot be evaluated].

3.2 Other relevant biological data

(a) *Experimental systems*

The oral LD_{50}'s of diglycidyl resorcinol ether in mice, rabbits and rats are 0.98, 1.24 and 2.57 g/kg bw, respectively. I.p. LD_{50}'s in mice and rats are 243 and 178 mg/kg bw.

Air saturated with diglycidyl resorcinol ether vapour was not lethal to mice and rats after 8 hours' exposure; but rabbits which received 7.2 g/kg bw by inhalation died. Repeated percutaneous applications of up to a total of 1.2 g diglycidyl resorcinol ether also caused death in rabbits. It caused irritation to the eyes and skin (Hine et al., 1958).

In monkeys, a once monthly i.v. injection of 100-200 mg/kg bw diglycidyl resorcinol ether produced a progressive lowering of the leucocyte count (Hine & Rowe, 1963). It produced a 27% inhibition of the growth of Walker carcinoma in rats (Hendry et al., 1951).

(b) Man

Diglycidyl resorcinol ether produces severe burns on contact with the skin, and skin sensitization has occurred in a limited number of cases (Hine & Rowe, 1963).

3.3 Observations in man

No data were available to the Working Group.

4. Comments on Data Reported and Evaluation

4.1 Animal data

Diglycidyl resorcinol ether was reported in a preliminary communication to be carcinogenic in mice by skin application and in rats by subcutaneous injection. No carcinogenic effect was observed in a further long-term skin application study in mice. No evaluation can be made.

4.2 Human data

No case reports or epidemiological studies were available to the Working Group.

5. References

Hawley, G.G., ed. (1971) The Condensed Chemical Dictionary, 8th ed., New York, Van Nostrand-Reinhold, p. 927

Hendry, J.A., Homer, R.F., Rose, F.L. & Walpole, A.L. (1951) Cytotoxic agents. II. Bis-epoxides and related compounds. Brit. J. Pharmacol., 6, 235-255

Hine, C.H. & Rowe, V.K. (1963) Resorcinol diglycidyl ether. In: Patty, F.A., ed., Industrial Hygiene and Toxicology, 2nd ed., Vol. 2, New York, Interscience, pp. 1648-1649

Hine, C.H., Kodama, J.K., Anderson, H.H., Simonson, D.W. & Wellington, J.S. (1958) The toxicology of epoxy resins. Arch. industr. Hlth, 17, 129-144

Lee, H. & Neville, K. (1967) Handbook of Epoxy Resins, San Francisco, McGraw-Hill, pp. 4-59

McCammon, C.J., Kotin, P. & Falk, H.L. (1957) The carcinogenic potency of certain diepoxides. Proc. Amer. Ass. Cancer Res., 2, 229-230

Van Duuren, B.L., Orris, L. & Nelson, N. (1965) Carcinogenicity of epoxides, lactones and peroxy compounds. II. J. nat. Cancer Inst., 35, 707-717

Werner, E.G.G. & Farenhorst, E. (1948) Glycidyl ethers. I. The synthesis of diglycidyl ethers. Rec. Trav. chim., 67, 438-441

EPICHLOROHYDRIN*

1. Chemical and Physical Data

1.1 Synonyms and trade names

Chem. Abstr. Reg. Serial No.: 106-89-8

Chem. Abstr. Name: Chloromethyl oxirane

1-Chloro-2,3-epoxypropane; 3-chloro-1,2-epoxypropane; (chloromethyl)ethylene oxide; 2-(chloromethyl)oxirane; chloropropylene oxide; γ-chloropropylene oxide; 3-chloro-1,2-propylene oxide; epichlorhydrin; α-epichlorohydrin; (DL)-α-epichlorohydrin; 1,2-epoxy-3-chloropropane; 2,3-epoxypropyl chloride

SKEKhG

1.2 Chemical formula and molecular weight

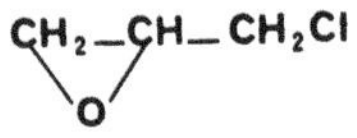

$$CH_2-CH-CH_2Cl$$
$$\diagdown O \diagup$$

C_3H_5ClO Mol. wt.: 92.5

1.3 Chemical and physical properties

(a) Description: Colourless liquid

(b) Boiling-point: 116.2°C

(c) Melting-point: -25.6°C

(d) Density: d_4^{20} 1.1812; d_4^{25} 1.1750

(e) Refractive index: n_D^{25} 1.4359

(f) Solubility: Miscible with water (6.4% by wt at 20°C); miscible with ethanol, diethyl ether and chlorinated aliphatic hydrocarbon solvents; immiscible with petroleum hydrocarbons

---

*Considered by the Working Group, February 1976

(g) <u>Stability</u>: Hydrolysis is slow at room temperature but is accelerated by heat or traces of acid.

(h) <u>Reactivity</u>: Reactions with active hydrogen compounds (e.g., alcohols, amines) normally occur at the more reactive epoxide site of epichlorohydrin, although reactions involving the chlorine are also known to occur. It reacts with 4-(4'-nitrobenzyl)pyridine (Preussmann *et al.*, 1969).

1.4 Technical products and impurities

Commercial specifications for a product sold by one US manufacturer are a minimum of 98.0% wt purity and a maximum of 0.2% wt water. Specifications for a product sold in Japan are a purity of over 98% and less than 0.1% water.

2. Production, Use, Occurrence and Analysis

For important background information on this section, see preamble, p. 19

2.1 Production and use

Synthesis of epichlorohydrin was carried out by Berthelot in 1854 by treatment of a crude glycerol dichlorohydrin mixture with alkali (Lichtenwalter & Riesser, 1964). It is produced commercially by the high-temperature chlorination of propylene to allyl chloride, followed by chlorohydrination with hypochlorous acid to yield a mixture of isomeric glycerol chlorohydrins, which are subsequently treated with alkali to yield epichlorohydrin.

In the US, small-scale production of epichlorohydrin started in about 1937 and large-scale production in 1949, in connection with the first synthetic glycerin plant. Production by two companies in 1973 was about 156.5 million kg. Epichlorohydrin has been produced commercially in Japan since 1966; production in 1974 is estimated to have been approximately 41 million kg. It is also known to be produced by one or more companies in the following countries: Czechoslovakia, France, Federal Republic of Germany, German Democratic Republic, The Netherlands, UK and USSR.

The estimated 1973 US consumption of epichlorohydrin was distributed as follows: synthetic glycerin, 46.4%; unmodified epoxy resins, 38.8%; epichlorohydrin elastomers, 1.7%; other products, 9.3%; exports, 3.8%. The consumption pattern in Japan is believed to be similar to that in the US.

In the production of synthetic glycerin, epichlorohydrin is hydrolysed to the α-monochlorohydrin, which is converted to glycerin with alkali. In the preparation of unmodified epoxy resins, epichlorohydrin is reacted with bisphenol-A to produce epoxy-terminated resins which are subsequently cured by further reaction with other chemicals (e.g., amines or anhydrides).

Epichlorohydrin elastomers represent a relatively small proportion of epichlorohydrin-derived products, but such elastomers are used when resistance to ozone, oil and solvents and impermeability to gases are required. Other products produced from epichlorohydrin, most of them in relatively small amounts, include glycidyl ethers, some types of modified epoxy resins, wet-strength resins for the paper industry and water treatment resins.

It has been used to crosslink starch in food and industrial uses. The food grade product is subject in some countries to regulations regarding the residue of epichlorohydrin and/or its hydrolysis products.

Permissible levels of epichlorohydrin in the working environment have been established in various countries (Winell, 1975). The threshold limit value in the US is 19 mg/m^3 (15 ppm); the maximum allowable concentration in the USSR is 1 mg/m^3.

2.2 Occurrence

No data were available to the Working Group.

2.3 Analysis

Epichlorohydrin can be determined volumetrically (Swan, 1954). A method for its colorimetric determination in air samples with chromotropic acid after periodate oxidation has been described (Jaraczewska & Kaszper, 1967). It has also been determined (with a limit of detection of 0.3%) in aqueous solutions after extraction with carbon tetrachloride by measurement of the absorbance at 1273 cm^{-1} (Adamek & Peterka, 1972). See also section 'General Remarks on the Substances Considered', p. 29.

3. Biological Data Relevant to the Evaluation of Carcinogenic Risk to Man

3.1 Carcinogenicity and related studies in animals

(a) Skin application

Mouse: Of 40 90-day old C3H mice painted thrice weekly with one 'brushful' of undiluted epichlorohydrin on the clipped dorsal skin for life, 30 were alive at 17 months, and 1 survived for 25 months. No tumours were observed (Weil et al., 1963).

Fifty 6-8-week old female ICR/Ha Swiss mice received 2 mg epichlorohydrin in 0.1 ml acetone thrice weekly on the clipped dorsal skin. The duration of the experiment was 580 days, and the median survival time, 506 days. No skin tumours were observed (Van Duuren et al., 1974).

In an initiation-promotion experiment, 30 mice received single doses of 2 mg epichlorohydrin in 0.1 ml acetone on the skin, followed 2 weeks later by thrice weekly skin applications of 2.5 µg phorbol myristate acetate in 0.1 ml acetone for the duration of the experiment (385 days). Nine mice developed skin papillomas (the first observed after 92 days), and 1 mouse developed a skin carcinoma. Of 30 control animals treated with phorbol myristate acetate alone, 3 developed papillomas (the first observed after 224 days). No tumours occurred in 30 solvent-treated controls (Van Duuren et al., 1974).

(b) Subcutaneous and/or intramuscular administration

Mouse: Of 50 6-week old female ICR/Ha Swiss mice which received weekly s.c. injections of 1 mg epichlorohydrin in 0.1 ml tricaprylin, 2 developed local sarcomas after 300 days (the first after 126 days). In earlier experiments the vehicle had proved to be non-carcinogenic (Van Duuren et al., 1972).

Of 50 6-8-week old female ICR/Ha Swiss mice given weekly s.c. injections of 1 mg epichlorohydrin in 0.05 ml tricaprylin for the duration of the experiment (580 days), 6 developed local sarcomas and 1 had a local adenocarcinoma. The median survival time was 486 days. One local sarcoma occurred in 50 tricaprylin-injected controls ($P<0.05$) (Van Duuren et al., 1974).

(c) Intraperitoneal administration

Mouse: Of 30 female ICR/Ha Swiss mice given weekly i.p. injections of 1 mg epichlorohydrin in 0.05 ml tricaprylin for the duration of the experiment (450 days), 11 developed papillary tumours of the lung. Of 30 controls treated with tricaprylin alone, 10 developed tumours of the lung (Van Duuren et al., 1974).

3.2 Other relevant biological data

(a) Experimental systems

The i.p. LD_{50}'s of epichlorohydrin range from 0.12-0.17 g/kg bw for rats, mice, guinea-pigs and rabbits. Oral LD_{50}'s in mice and rats are 0.24 and 0.26 g/kg, respectively. The LD_{50} following percutaneous administration to rabbits is 0.76 g/kg bw. The median time to death of mice inhaling an air-vapour mixture containing 72 g/m^3 epichlorohydrin was 9 minutes (Laurence et al., 1972).

Epichlorohydrin can cause central nervous depression and irritation of the respiratory tract; death is generally due to depression of the respiratory centre (Hine & Rowe, 1963). Nephrotoxicity is a cumulative effect of epichlorohydrin poisoning (Hine & Rowe, 1963; Pallade et al., 1968); renal insufficiency occurred within 24-48 hours in approximately 80% of rats that had been given 125 mg/kg bw of the compound (Pallade et al., 1968). It produces extreme irritation when tested intradermally, dermally or intraocularly in rabbits (Laurence et al., 1972).

In a 12-week subacute toxicity test in rats injected intraperitoneally with epichlorohydrin, treatment led to a dose-related decrease in haemoglobin values; with doses of 0.056 g/kg bw an increase in segmented neutrophils was seen; a reduction in the proportion of lymphocytes occurred at doses of 0.022 and 0.056 g/kg bw (Laurence et al., 1972). An increased leucocyte count was observed in animals which were exposed chronically to vapours of epichlorohydrin in air at concentrations of 2 mg/m^3 (Fomin, 1966). The maximum tolerated dose in a 13-week subacute study in rats following oral administration of epichlorohydrin was 45 mg/kg bw/day (Oser et al., 1975).

Repeated oral administration of 15 mg/kg bw epichlorohydrin produced reversible infertility in male rats within 7 days: fertility was restored after dosing had been discontinued for approximately 1 week (Hahn, 1970).

It produced a 27% inhibition of the growth of Walker carcinoma in rats (Hendry *et al.*, 1951).

Epichlorohydrin in ethanol produced reverse mutations in *Escherichia coli* strain B/r (Strauss & Okubo, 1960); and a 0.15 M aqueous solution induced reverse mutations in macroconidia of the purple, adenine-requiring mutant 38701 of *Neurospora crassa* after 30 minutes (Kølmark & Giles, 1955). Recessive lethal mutations have been obtained in *Drosophila melanogaster* after treatment with epichlorohydrin (Rapoport, 1948).

A dose of 150 mg/kg bw epichlorohydrin administered by i.p. injection did not induce dominant lethal mutations in ICR/Ha Swiss mice (Epstein *et al.*, 1972).

(b) Man

Fomin (1966) found that exposure to epichlorohydrin at a concentration of 0.3 mg/m^3, which represents a threshold value for the smell of that substance for the most sensitive human subjects, produced changes in the electroencephalogram pattern, whereas a concentration of 0.2 mg/m^3 was inactive.

Several cases of severe skin burns have resulted from local contact with epichlorohydrin (Hine & Rowe, 1963). One case of severe epichlorohydrin poisoning occurred in a 39-year old laboratory assistant: initial irritation of the eyes and throat was followed by chronic asthmatic bronchitis; successive biopsies established a high degree of fatty infiltration of the liver (Schultz, 1964).

3.3 Observations in man

No data were available to the Working Group.

4. Comments on Data Reported and Evaluation[1]

4.1 Animal data

Epichlorohydrin is carcinogenic in mice by subcutaneous injection: it produced local sarcomas. It was active as an initiator in a two-stage skin carcinogenesis study in mice.

4.2 Human data

No case reports or epidemiological studies were available to the Working Group.

---

[1] See also the section 'Animal Data in Relation to the Evaluation of Risk to Man' in the introduction to this volume, p. 17.

5. References

Adamek, P. & Peterka, V. (1972) Determination of epichlorohydrin in the reaction mixture after its hydrolysis. Veda Vyzk. Potravin. Prum., 23, 135-141

Epstein, S.S., Arnold, E., Andrea, J., Bass, W. & Bishop, Y. (1972) Detection of chemical mutagens by the dominant lethal assay in the mouse. Toxicol. appl. Pharmacol., 23, 288-325

Fomin, A.P. (1966) Biological effect of epichlorohydrin and its hygienic significance as an atmospheric contamination factor. Gig. i Sanit., 31, 7-11

Hahn, J.D. (1970) Post-testicular antifertility effect of epichlorohydrin and 2,3-epoxypropanol. Nature (Lond.), 226, 87

Hendry, J.A., Homer, R.F., Rose, F.L. & Walpole, A.L. (1951) Cytotoxic agents. II. Bis-epoxides and related compounds. Brit. J. Pharmacol., 6, 235-255

Hine, C.H. & Rowe, V.K. (1963) Epichlorohydrin. In: Patty, F.A., ed., Industrial Hygiene and Toxicology, 2nd ed., Vol. 2, New York, Interscience, pp. 1622-1625

Jaraczewska, W. & Kaszper, W. (1967) Determination of epichlorohydrin in the air. Med. Pracy, 18, 169-176

Kølmark, G. & Giles, N.H. (1955) Comparative studies of monoepoxides as inducers of reverse mutations in Neurospora. Genetics, 40, 890-902

Laurence, W.H., Malik, M., Turner, J.E. & Autian, J. (1972) Toxicity profile of epichlorohydrin. J. pharm. Sci., 61, 1712-1717

Lichtenwalter, G.D. & Riesser, G.H. (1964) Chlorohydrins. In: Kirk, R.E. & Othmer, D.F., eds, Encyclopedia of Chemical Technology, 2nd ed., Vol. 5, New York, John Wiley and Sons, pp. 318-324

Oser, B.L., Morgareidge, K., Cox, G.E. & Carson, S. (1975) Short-term toxicity of ethylene chlorohydrin (ECH) in rats, dogs and monkeys. Fd Cosmet. Toxicol., 13, 313-315

Pallade, S., Dorobantu, M. & Gabrielescu, E. (1968) Insuffisance rénale aiguë dans l'intoxication par l'épichlorhydrine. Arch. Mal. prof., 29, 679-688

Preussmann, R., Schneider, H. & Epple, F. (1969) Untersuchungen zum Nachweis alkylierender Agentien. II. Der Nachweis verschiedener Klassen alkylierender Agentien mit einer Modifikation der Farbreaktion mit 4-(4'-Nitrobenzyl)pyridin (NBP). Arzneimittelforsch., 19, 1059-1073

Rapoport, I.A. (1948) Action of ethylene oxide, glycidol and glycols on gene mutation. Dokl. Akad. Nauk SSR, 60, 469-472

Schultz, C. (1964) Fettleber und chronisch-asthmoide Bronchitis nach Inhalation eines Farbenlösungsmittels (Epichlorhydrin). Dtsch. med. Wschr., 89, 1342-1344

Strauss, B. & Okubo, S. (1960) Protein synthesis and the induction of mutations in *Escherichia coli* by alkylating agents. J. Bact., 79, 464-473

Swan, J.D. (1954) Determination of epoxides with sodium sulfite. Analyt. Chem., 26, 878-880

Van Duuren, B.L., Katz, C., Goldschmidt, B.M., Frenkel, K. & Sivak, A. (1972) Carcinogenicity of halo-ethers. II. Structure-activity relationships of analogs of bis(chloromethyl)ether. J. nat. Cancer Inst., 48, 1431-1439

Van Duuren, B.L., Goldschmidt, B.M., Katz, C., Seidmann, I. & Paul, J.S. (1974) Carcinogenic activity of alkylating agents. J. nat. Cancer Inst., 53, 695-700

Weil, C.S., Condra, N., Haun, C. & Striegel, J.A. (1963) Experimental carcinogenicity and acute toxicity of representative epoxides. Amer. industr. Hyg. Ass. J., 24, 305-325

Winell, M.A. (1975) An international comparison of hygienic standards for chemicals in the work environment. Ambio, 4, 34-36

1-EPOXYETHYL-3,4-EPOXYCYCLOHEXANE*

1. Chemical and Physical Data

1.1 Synonyms and trade names

Chem. Abstr. Reg. Serial No.: 106-87-6

Chem. Abstr. Name: 3-Oxiranyl-7-oxabicyclo(4.1.0)heptane

1,2-Epoxy-4-(epoxyethyl)cyclohexane; 3-(epoxyethyl)-7-oxabicyclo-(4.1.0)heptane; 4-(epoxyethyl)-7-oxabicyclo(4.1.0)heptane; 3-(1,2-epoxyethyl)-7-oxabicyclo(4.1.0)heptane; 4-(1,2-epoxyethyl)-7-oxabicyclo(4.1.0)heptane; vinylcyclohexane diepoxide; vinyl-cyclohexene diepoxide; 4-vinylcyclohexene diepoxide; 4-vinyl-1-cyclohexene diepoxide; 4-vinyl-1,2-cyclohexene diepoxide; vinyl cyclohexene dioxide; vinylcyclohexene dioxide; 4-vinylcyclohexene dioxide; 1-vinyl-3-cyclohexene dioxide; 4-vinyl-1-cyclohexene dioxide

Chissonox 206; Unox Epoxide 206

1.2 Chemical formula and molecular weight

$C_8H_{12}O_2$ Mol. wt: 140.2

1.3 Chemical and physical properties

(a) <u>Description</u>: Colourless liquid

(b) <u>Boiling-point</u>: 227°C at 760 mm; 110-113°C at 20 mm

(c) <u>Freezing-point</u>: Sets to a glass at -55°C

(d) <u>Density</u>: d_{20}^{20} 1.0986

---

*Considered by the Working Group, February 1976

(e) <u>Refractive index</u>: n_D^{20} 1.4787

(f) <u>Spectroscopy data</u>: Infra-red epoxide band at 1250 cm^{-1}

(g) <u>Solubility</u>: Miscible with water (18.3% w/w) at 20°C

(h) <u>Stability</u>: Slowly hydrolysed in water

(i) <u>Reactivity</u>: Reacts with active hydrogen compounds (e.g., alcohols, amines)

1.4 Technical products and impurities

One grade of 1-epoxyethyl-3,4-epoxycyclohexane available in the US has an epoxy equivalent of 74-78 (Anon., 1964).

2. Production, Use, Occurrence and Analysis

For important background information on this section, see preamble, p. 19.

2.1 Production and use

1-Epoxyethyl-3,4-epoxycyclohexane can be prepared by peracetic acid epoxidization of 4-vinylcyclohexane (Wallace, 1964).

It has been produced commercially by one US manufacturer for about 20 years, but no data on US production, imports or exports are available.

The compound is used as a reactive diluent for other diepoxides and for epoxy resins derived from bisphenol-A and epichlorohydrin. It has also been proposed for use as a chemical intermediate (e.g., for condensation with dicarboxylic acids) and as a monomer (e.g., for preparation of polyglycols containing unreacted epoxy groups or for homo-polymerization to a three dimensional resin) (Anon., 1964).

2.2 Occurrence

No data were available to the Working Group.

2.3 Analysis

Gas chromatography and infra-red spectroscopy have been used. See also section 'General Remarks on the Substances Considered', p. 29.

3. Biological Data Relevant to the Evaluation of Carcinogenic Risk to Man

3.1 Carcinogenicity and related studies in animals

(a) Skin application

Mouse: Repeated skin applications of 16 mg of a commercial sample of 1-epoxyethyl-3,4-epoxycyclohexane in acetone 5 times weekly for 12 months produced skin tumours in 11/20 male albino mice; 9 of these had squamous-cell carcinomas and/or sarcomas. The last mouse died 21 months after the start of treatment; no control data were reported (Hendry et al., 1951). In two other studies, 1/20 and 4/18 C57Bl or C3H mice developed skin tumours after applications of a 10% solution in acetone and total doses of 70 and 78 mg (Kotin & Falk, 1963; Weil et al., 1963) [Control data were given for neither of the above studies].

Of 30 8-week old male Swiss ICR/Ha mice painted on the clipped dorsal skin with 0.1 ml of a 10% solution in benzene thrice weekly, 14 developed skin tumours; 9 of these had squamous-cell carcinomas; the mean survival time was 326 days. Among 150 benzene-treated mice, skin tumours occurred in 11, 1 of which had a squamous-cell carcinoma. Of 207 untreated mice, 13 had skin tumours; 1 of these had a squamous-cell carcinoma (Van Duuren et al., 1963) [$P<0.001$].

(b) Intraperitoneal administration

Rat: Of 10 male and 4 female stock albino rats given twice weekly i.p. injections of 250 mg/kg bw 1-epoxy-3,4-epoxycyclohexane in arachis oil for 10 weeks, 1 male developed a sarcoma in the peritoneal cavity after 7 months. No other tumours occurred in other rats surviving 21 months. No data were reported for arachis oil-injected controls (Hendry et al., 1951).

3.2 Other relevant biological data

In rats, the oral LD_{50} of 1-epoxy-3,4-epoxycyclohexane is 2.83 g/kg bw; in rabbits, the percutaneous LD_{50} is 0.68 mg/kg bw (Weil et al., 1963). The 4-hour inhalational LC_{50} in rats was 4580 mg/m^3 (800 ppm); death occurred soon after exposure (Hine & Rowe, 1963).

This compound causes acute respiratory-tract irritation and congestion of the lungs. It produces redness and swelling compatible with a first-degree burn on the clipped skin of rabbits. Treated rats showed focal necrosis of the thymus, and the leucocyte count fell by more than 60% during the first 4 days (Kodama et al., 1961). Both Kodama et al. (1961) and Hine & Rowe (1963) report testicular atrophy in some of the animals that had been exposed to this compound.

This epoxide causes 94% inhibition of the growth of Walker carcinoma in rats (Hendry et al., 1951).

3.3 Observations in man

No data were available to the Working Group.

4. Comments on Data Reported and Evaluation[1]

4.1 Animal data

1-Epoxyethyl-3,4-epoxycyclohexane is carcinogenic in mice by skin application: it produced squamous-cell skin carcinomas.

4.2 Human data

No case reports or epidemiological studies were available to the Working Group.

---

[1] See also the section 'Animal Data in Relation to the Evaluation of Risk to Man' in the introduction to this volume, p. 17.

5. References

Anon. (1964) *Bakelite Epoxy Resin ERL-4206*, Technical Bulletin, 4-1456, New York, Union Carbide Co.

Hendry, J.A., Homer, R.F., Rose, F.L. & Walpole, A.L. (1951) Cytotoxic agents. II. Bis-epoxides and related compounds. *Brit. J. Pharmacol.*, 6, 235-255

Hine, C.H. & Rowe, V.K. (1963) *Vinylcyclohexene dioxide*. In: Patty, F.A., ed., *Industrial Hygiene and Toxicology*, 2nd ed., Vol. 2, New York, Interscience, pp. 1651-1652

Kodama, J.K., Guzman, R.J., Dunlap, M.K., Loquvam, G.S., Lima, R. & Hine, C.H. (1961) Some effects of epoxy compounds on the blood. *Arch. environm. Hlth*, 2, 56-67

Kotin, P. & Falk, H.L. (1963) Organic peroxides, hydrogen peroxide, epoxides and neoplasia. *Radiation Res. Suppl.*, 3, 193-211

Van Duuren, B.L., Nelson, N., Orris, L., Palmes, E.D. & Schmitt, F.L. (1963) Carcinogenicity of epoxides, lactones and peroxy compounds. *J. nat. Cancer Inst.*, 31, 41-55

Wallace, J.G. (1964) *Epoxidation*. In: Kirk, R.E. & Othmer, D.F., eds, *Encyclopedia of Chemical Technology*, 2nd ed., Vol. 8, New York, John Wiley and Sons, pp. 249-265

Weil, C.S., Condra, N., Haun, C. & Striegel, J.A. (1963) Experimental carcinogenicity and acute toxicity of representative epoxides. *Amer. industr. Hyg. Ass. J.*, 24, 305-325

3,4-EPOXY-6-METHYLCYCLOHEXYLMETHYL-3,4-EPOXY-6-METHYLCYCLOHEXANE CARBOXYLATE*

1. Chemical and Physical Data

1.1 Synonyms and trade names

Chem. Abstr. Reg. Serial No.: 141-37-7

Chem. Abstr. Name: 4-Methyl-7-oxabicyclo(4.1.0)heptane-3-carboxylic acid, 4-methyl-7-oxabicylo(4.1.0)hept-3-yl methyl ester

α-Dicyclodiepoxycarboxyl-3,4-epoxy-6-methylcyclohexylmethyl-3,4-epoxy-6-methylcyclohexenecarboxylate; 3,4-epoxy-6-methylcyclohexanecarboxylic acid, (3,4-epoxy-6-methylcyclohexylmethyl)ester; 3,4-epoxy-6-methylcyclohexylmethyl-3,4-epoxy-6-methylcyclohexanecarboxylate; 3,4-epoxy-6-methylcyclohexylmethyl-3',4'-epoxy-6'-methylcyclohexane carboxylate; 4,5-epoxy-2-methylcyclohexylmethyl-4,5-epoxy-2-methylcyclohexanecarboxylate; 6-methyl-3,4-epoxycyclohexylmethyl 6-methyl-3,4-epoxycyclohexane carboxylate; (6-methyl-3,4-epoxycyclohexyl)methyl 6-methyl-3,4-epoxycyclohexanecarboxylate; 4-methyl-7-oxabicyclo(4.1.0)heptane-3-methanol-4-methyl-7-oxabicyclo-(4.1.0)heptane-3-carboxylate

Chissonox 201; EP 201; Epoxide 201; Unox 201; Unox Epoxide 201

1.2 Chemical formula and molecular weight

$C_{16}H_{24}O_4$ Mol. wt: 280.4

---

*Considered by the Working Group, February 1976

1.3 Chemical and physical properties

(a) Description: Liquid

(b) Boiling-point: 123-135°C at 0.08 mm; 185-186°C at 3 mm; 215°C at 5 mm

(c) Density: d_{20}^{20} 1.121

(d) Refractive index: n_D^{25} 1.4937; n_D^{26} 1.4861; n_D^{30} 1.4822

(e) Solubility: Miscible with water (0.3% w/w) and acetone

1.4 Technical products and impurities

No data were available to the Working Group.

2. Production, Use, Occurrence and Analysis

For important background information on this section, see preamble, p. 19.

2.1 Production and use

This chemical was produced in the US by one company until about 1965 for use in the manufacture of cured resins by reaction with a variety of curing agents. It is believed to have been replaced in these applications by the corresponding chemical which lacks the methyl groups on each of the cyclohexyl rings.

2.2 Occurrence

No data were available to the Working Group.

2.3 Analysis

This chemical can be detected by paper chromatography, with a limit of detection of 10 µg (Novak, 1968). See also section 'General Remarks on the Substances Considered', p. 29.

3. Biological Data Relevant to the Evaluation of Carcinogenic Risk to Man

3.1 Carcinogenicity and related studies in animals

Skin application

Mouse: Groups of 30-40 13-week old C3H mice, 21 52-week old 1C3FL and 23 52-week old C31FL mice were painted on the clipped dorsal skin thrice weekly with one 'brushful' of the undiluted substance (u), or a mixture of 50 parts with 50 parts dodecane (do), for life (see table). The numbers of mice that developed skin tumours (papillomas and carcinomas) in relation to the numbers of animals alive at the appearance of the first tumour were as follows:

Strain	Concentration	No. of mice alive at the appearance of first tumour	Total nos of mice with skin tumours	
			Papillomas	Carcinomas
C3H	u	15	9	3
C3H	u	39	20	9
C3H	u	21	14	7
C3H	u purified	37	29	21
1C3F1	u	18	13	6
C31F1	u	9	7	1
C3H	do	37	9	6

No tumours developed in 2 groups of 27 and 28 C3H mice painted with a 5% solution of the compound in acetone and surviving 17 or more months (Weil et al., 1963).

Of 30 8-week old female ICR/Ha Swiss mice painted on the clipped dorsal skin thrice weekly with approximately 0.1 ml of a 10% solution in acetone for life, 11 animals developed skin carcinomas, the first of which was observed after 544 days, and 11 had skin keratoacanthomas. The median survival time was longer than the 544 days which constituted the duration of the experiment. No skin tumours developed in 120 control animals painted with acetone (Van Duuren et al., 1967).

3.2 Other relevant biological data

The oral LD_{50} in rats is 5.51 g/kg bw. Rats exposed to a mixture in air saturated at $17^{\circ}C$ survived a 4-hour exposure, but 5/6 died following an 8-hour exposure. Rabbits survived single skin applications of 11 g/kg bw (Weil et al., 1963). The substance caused faint erythema on rabbit skin (Hine & Rowe, 1963).

3.3 Observations in man

No data were available to the Working Group.

4. Comments on Data Reported and Evaluation[1]

4.1 Animal data

3,4-Epoxy-6-methylcyclohexylmethyl-3,4-epoxy-6-methylcyclohexane carboxylate is carcinogenic in mice by skin application: it produced skin carcinomas.

4.2 Human data

No case reports or epidemiological studies were available to the Working Group.

---

[1]See also the section 'Animal Data in Relation to the Evaluation of Risk to Man' in the introduction to this volume, p. 17.

5. References

Hine, C.H. & Rowe, V.K. (1963) Epoxide 201. In: Patty, F.A., ed., Industrial Hygiene and Toxicology, 2nd ed., Vol. 2, New York, Interscience, pp. 1625-1626

Novak, J. (1968) Über die Papierchromatographie cycloaliphatischer Epoxide. J. Chromat., 35, 83-91

Van Duuren, B.L., Langseth, L., Goldschmidt, B.M. & Orris, L. (1967) Carcinogenicity of epoxides, lactones and peroxy compounds. VI. Structure and carcinogenic activity. J. nat. Cancer Inst., 39, 1217-1228

Weil, C.S., Condra, N., Haun, C. & Striegel, J.A. (1963) Experimental carcinogenicity and acute toxicity of representative epoxides. Amer. industr. Hyg. Ass. J., 24, 305-325

CIS-9,10-EPOXYSTEARIC ACID*

1. Chemical and Physical Data

1.1 Synonyms and trade names

Chem. Abstr. Reg. Serial No.: 2443-39-2

Chem. Abstr. Name: cis-3-Octyl-oxiraneoctanoic acid

cis-9,10-Epoxyoctadecanoic acid; cis-9,10-epoxy octadecanoate; epoxyoleic acid

1.2 Chemical formula and molecular weight

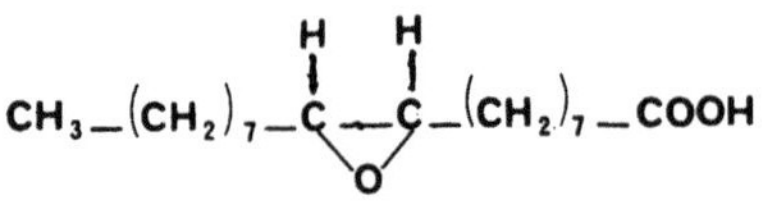

$$CH_3-(CH_2)_7-\overset{H}{\underset{\diagdown O \diagup}{C}}-\overset{H}{C}-(CH_2)_7-COOH$$

$C_{18}H_{34}O_3$ Mol. wt: 298.5

1.3 Chemical and physical properties

(a) Description: Colourless platelets (from acetone)

(b) Melting-point: 59.5-59.8°C

(c) Solubility: Soluble in ethanol, ether, chloroform and ethyl acetate

1.4 Technical products and impurities

No data were available to the Working Group.

2. Production, Use, Occurrence and Analysis

2.1 Production and use

cis-9,10-Epoxystearic acid can be prepared from oleic acid by reaction with perbenzoic acid (Swern et al., 1944) or by reaction with hypoiodous

---

*Considered by the Working Group, February 1976

acid followed by treatment of the resulting iodohydroxy acid with alcoholic potassium hydroxide (Rankov & Ivanova, 1968). It is manufactured only in laboratory quantities for research purposes.

2.2 Occurrence

The glyceride of *cis*-9,10-epoxystearic acid is a constituent of the oil of sal nuts from the tree *Shorea robusta* (Bringi et al., 1972) and is found in some malvaceous seed oils (Hassan El Mallah et al., 1966). The acid has been detected at levels of up to 0.5% in a number of sunflower seed oil samples after prolonged storage (Mikolajczak et al., 1968).

2.3 Analysis

The methyl ester of *cis*-9,10-epoxystearic acid can be analysed by gas-liquid chromatography (Mikolajczak et al., 1968). See also section 'General Remarks on the Substances Considered', p. 29.

3. Biological Data Relevant to the Evaluation of Carcinogenic Risk to Man

3.1 Carcinogenicity and related studies in animals

(a) Skin application

Mouse: Of 30 8-week old male ICR/Ha Swiss mice painted with about 0.1 ml of a 1% solution of *cis*-9,10-epoxystearic acid in acetone thrice weekly on the clipped dorsal skin for life, 3 developed skin papillomas. The median survival time was 165 days. Of 90 acetone-treated controls, 8 mice had papillomas (Van Duuren et al., 1963). In a similar experiment, 30 8-week old female ICR/Ha Swiss mice were painted on the clipped dorsal skin thrice weekly with approximately 0.1 ml of a 10% solution of *cis*-9,10-epoxystearic acid in acetone. Half of the animals were alive when the experiment was terminated after 539 days. No skin tumours were observed (Van Duuren et al., 1967a).

(b) Subcutaneous and/or intramuscular administration

Mouse: Two groups of 50 and 30 8-week old female ICR/Ha Swiss mice were given weekly s.c. injections of 0.1 or 10 mg *cis*-9,10-epoxystearic acid in 0.05 ml tricaprylin. The median survival periods were 525 and

301 days, respectively, and the durations of the experiments were 590 and 530 days, respectively. No local tumours were observed (Van Duuren et al., 1966).

Three groups of 10 8-week old female BALB/c mice received twice weekly s.c. injections of 1.0, 0.5 or 0.005 mg cis-9,10-epoxystearic acid in 0.1 ml tricaprylin for 57 or 40 weeks. Eighteen animals were alive at 18 months, and 1 animal in each group developed a local sarcoma. A further 3 groups of 15 female CFW (Swiss-Webster) mice were treated as above for 41 weeks with doses of 1.0, 0.5 and 0.005 mg cis-9,10-epoxystearic acid in 0.1 ml tricaprylin. Twenty animals were alive at 18 months, and 3 mice (2 in the median dose group and 1 in the low dose group) developed local sarcomas. In a control group of 10 BALB/c mice treated with tricaprylin, 1/5 animals alive at 18 months developed a local sarcoma. No local tumours were observed in 21 control CFW mice injected with the vehicle and surviving 18 months (Swern et al., 1970).

Rat: Twenty 6-week old female Sprague-Dawley rats were given weekly s.c. injections of 100 mg cis-9,10-epoxystearic acid in 0.2 ml tricaprylin. The median survival time was 505 days, at which time the experiment was terminated. No local sarcomas were observed (Van Duuren et al., 1967b).

3.2 Other relevant biological data

No data were available to the Working Group.

3.3 Observations in man

No data were available to the Working Group.

4. Comments on Data Reported and Evaluation

4.1 Animal data

cis-9,10-Epoxystearic acid has been tested in mice by skin application and in mice and rats by subcutaneous injection. The limited amount of data do not indicate that the compound is carcinogenic.

4.2 Human data

No case reports or epidemiological studies were available to the Working Group.

5. References

Bringi, N.V., Padley, F.B. & Timms, R.E. (1972) Fatty acid and triglyceride compositions of *Shorea robusta* fat : occurrence of *cis*-9,10-epoxystearic acid and threo-9,10-dihydroxystearic acid. Chem. & Indust., 20, 805-806

Hassan El Mallah, M.M., Souka, L.M. & Gad, A.M. (1966) Epoxy acids and epoxidized oils. I. Quantitative evaluation of naturally occurring epoxy fatty acids in some malvaceous seed oils. Fette, Seifen, Anstrichm., 68, 1028-1030

Mikolajczak, K.L., Freidinger, R.M., Smith, C.F., Jr & Wolff, I.A. (1968) Oxygenated fatty acids of oil from sunflower seeds after prolonged storage. Lipids, 3, 489-494

Rankov, D. & Ivanova, B. (1968) Addition of hypoiodous acid to unsaturated fatty acids under conditions employed in the rapid method for the determination of iodine value of fats according to Margosches. I. Oleic and elaidic acids. Fette, Siefen, Anstrichm., 70, 334-340

Swern, D., Findley, F.W. & Scanlan, J.T. (1944) Epoxidation of oleic acid, methyl oleate and oleyl alcohol with perbenzoic acid. J. Amer. chem. Soc., 66, 1925-1927

Swern, D., Wieder, R., McDonough, M., Meranze, D.R. & Shimkin, M.B. (1970) Investigation of fatty acids and derivates for carcinogenic activity. Cancer Res., 30, 1037-1046

Van Duuren, B.L., Nelson, N., Orris, L., Palmes, E.D. & Schmitt, F.L. (1963) Carcinogenicity of epoxides, lactones and peroxy compounds. J. nat. Cancer Inst., 31, 41-55

Van Duuren, B.L., Langseth, L., Orris, L., Teebor, G., Nelson, N. & Kuschner, M. (1966) Carcinogenicity of epoxides, lactones and peroxy compounds. IV. Tumor response in epithelial and connective tissue in mice and rats. J. nat. Cancer Inst., 37, 825-838

Van Duuren, B.L., Langseth, L., Goldschmidt, B.M. & Orris, L. (1967a) Carcinogenicity of epoxides, lactones and peroxy compounds. VI. Structure and carcinogenic activity. J. nat. Cancer Inst., 39, 1217-1228

Van Duuren, B.L., Langseth, L., Orris, L., Baden, M. & Kuschner, M. (1967b) Carcinogenicity of epoxides, lactones and peroxy compounds. V. Subcutaneous injection in rats. J. nat. Cancer Inst., 39, 1213-1216

ETHYLENE OXIDE*

1. Chemical and Physical Data

1.1 Synonyms and trade names

Chem. Abstr. Reg. Serial No.: 75-21-8

Chem. Abstr. Name: Oxirane

Dihydrooxirene; dimethylene oxide; 1,2-epoxyethane; ethyleneoxide; ETO; oxacyclopropane; oxane; oxidoethane; α,β-oxidoethane

1.2 Chemical formula and molecular weight

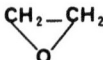

C_2H_4O Mol. wt: 44.1

1.3 Chemical and physical properties

(a) Description: Colourless, inflammable gas

(b) Boiling-point: 10.7°C

(c) Melting-point: -111°C

(d) Density: d_4^0 0.891; d_4^{20} 0.869

(e) Refractive index: n_D^7 1.3597

(f) Solubility: Soluble in water, ethanol and diethyl ether

(g) Volatility: The vapour pressure at 20°C is 1095 mm.

(h) Reactivity: Reacts with active hydrogen compounds (e.g., alcohols, amines and sulphydryl compounds) and with inorganic chloride in foods to form ethylene chlorohydrin (Ragelis et al., 1966; Wesley et al., 1965). It reacts with 4-(4'-nitrobenzyl)-pyridine (Preussmann et al., 1969).

---

*Considered by the Working Group, February 1976

1.4 Technical products and impurities

Ethylene oxide is available in cylinders or tank cars as technical and pure (99.7%) grades (Hawley, 1971). Specifications for a typical technical grade product are as follows: water, 0.03%; acetaldehyde, 0.01%; acetic acid, 0.002%; non-volatile residue, 0.1 g/l; residual odour, none. It is also available as a 10-80% pressurized or liquified gas formulated with carbon dioxide, trichlorofluoromethane or dichlorodifluoromethane to reduce fire hazards (US Environmental Protection Agency, 1973).

2. Production, Use, Occurrence and Analysis

For important background information on this section, see preamble, p. 19.

2.1 Production and use

Ethylene oxide was prepared in 1859 by Wurtz from ethylene chlorohydrin and potassium hydroxide (Stecher, 1968). This process was the principal method of manufacture until 1957 but has not been used in the US since 1972. All US production is now by the direct catalytic oxidation of ethylene with air or oxygen.

Ethylene oxide is produced in Argentina, Australia, Belgium, Brazil, Bulgaria, Canada, Czechoslovakia, Democratic German Republic, Federal Republic of Germany, France, India, Iran, Italy, Japan, Mexico, The Netherlands, North Korea, Poland, Romania, Spain, Sweden, Taiwan, UK, US and USSR.

Ethylene oxide was first produced commercially in the US in 1921 (US Tariff Commission, 1922). In March 1973, the 13 companies in the US and Puerto Rico had a total production of 1,892 million kg (US International Trade Commission, 1975).

It has been produced commercially in Japan since 1934 and is currently produced by five companies by the oxidation of ethylene. Total production in 1974 was 415 million kg. European production in 1972 has been estimated at 865 million kg.

The largest use for ethylene oxide is as an intermediate in the production of ethylene glycol, which is used mainly in anti-freeze products, and as an intermediate for polyethylene terephthalate polyester fibre and film production. It is also used in the manufacture of non-ionic surface-active agents, diethylene glycol, triethylene glycol, ethanolamines, choline and choline chloride and other organic chemicals.

It is estimated that 387 million kg ethylene oxide were used in Japan in 1974: 67% for ethylene glycol, 15% for surface-active agents, 6% for ethanolamine, 5% for glycol ethers, 2% for polyethylene glycol and 5% for other uses.

Ethylene oxide is registered in the US as a fungicide for treatment by fumigation of books; dental, pharmaceutical, medical and scientific equipment and supplies (glass, metals, plastics, rubber or textiles); drugs; leather; motor oil; paper; soil; bedding for experimental animals; clothing; furs; furniture; and transportation vehicles (jet aircraft, buses and railroad passenger cars) (US Environmental Protection Agency, 1973).

It has also been used to sterilize foodstuffs such as spices, cocoa, flour, dried egg powder, desiccated coconut, dried fruits and dehydrated vegetables (Wesley et al., 1965). It has been used to accelerate the maturing of tobacco leaves (Fishbein, 1969).

Permissible levels of ethylene oxide in the working environment have been established in various countries (Winell, 1975). The threshold limit value in the US is 90 mg/m^3 (50 ppm); the maximum allowable concentration in the USSR is 1 mg/m^3.

2.2 Occurrence

When bread in sealed plastic bags was treated with ethylene oxide, the initial concentration of the fumigant present in the atmosphere of the package was reduced by half immediately after the treatment; it was virtually negligible after 3 days (Buquet & Manchon, 1970; Manchon & Buquet, 1970). No ethylene oxide was found in fish or bone meals twelve hours after sterilizing, whereas meat meal contained traces of the fumigant 24 hours after treatment (Redaelli et al., 1967). In connection with the treatment of foods with ethylene oxide, it should be noted that this compound reacts with inorganic chloride in foods to form ethylene chlorohydrin (Ragelis et al., 1966; Wesley et al., 1965).

The ethylene oxide content of cigarette smoke was low in untreated cigarettes but increased with longer treatment time and/or higher concentrations of ethylene oxide. Similar levels were found in the smoke from commercial cigarettes from various countries (Austria, Federal Republic of Germany, Japan, UK and US) (Muramatsu *et al.*, 1968). In experiments with Austrian cigarettes, the particulate phase of the smoke was removed with a Cambridge filter, and the concentrations of ethylene oxide were found to be 0.02 μg/ml for untreated tobacco, 0.05 μg/ml for tobacco treated with 150 g ethylene oxide per m^3 and up to 0.3 μg/ml for tobacco exhaustively fumigated (Binder & Lindner, 1972). Commercial charcoal filters remove ethylene oxide from cigarette smoke (Muramatsu *et al.*, 1968).

Ethylene oxide is used in the US as a post-harvest fumigant for black walnut meats, copra and whole spices; residues of up to 50 mg/kg are permitted (US Code of Federal Regulations, 1974).

The use of ethylene oxide as a fumigant and its transformation into ethylene chlorohydrin have been reviewed (FAO/WHO, 1972). No tolerances were proposed for levels of ethylene oxide as ethylene chlorohydrin in food.

2.3 Analysis

Ethylene oxide can be determined by spectrophotometry (Pozzoli *et al.*, 1968) by colorimetry (Adler, 1965; Critchfield & Johnson, 1957; Gage, 1957) or volumetrically (Gunther, 1965; Hollingsworth & Waling, 1955; Lubatti, 1944; Swan, 1954). Gas chromatography of air samples and residues from fumigated materials has been used for foodstuffs, pharmaceuticals and surgical equipment (Adler, 1965; Ben-Yehoshua & Krinsky, 1968; Berck, 1965; Brown, 1970; Buquet & Manchon, 1970; Heuser & Scudamore, 1968, 1969; Kulkarni *et al.*, 1968; Manchon & Buquet, 1970). It can be determined in cigarette smoke by gas chromatography or mass spectrometry after conversion to ethylene chlorohydrin (Binder & Lindner, 1972; Muramatsu *et al.*, 1968) and in mixtures of lower olefin oxides and aldehydes by gas chromatography (Kaliberdo & Vaabel, 1967). The limits of detection by spectrophotometry and gas chromatography were generally of the order of 1 mg/kg.

For methods of analysis of ethylene oxide and associated residues in commodities fumigated with ethylene oxide see FAO/WHO (1972).

3. Biological Data Relevant to the Evaluation of Carcinogenic Risk to Man

3.1 Carcinogenicity and related studies in animals

(a) Skin application

Mouse: Thirty 8-week old female ICR/Ha Swiss mice were painted thrice weekly on the clipped dorsal skin with approximately 0.1 ml of a 10% solution of ethylene oxide in acetone for life. The median survival time was 493 days; no skin tumours were observed (Van Duuren et al., 1965).

(b) Subcutaneous and/or intramuscular administration

Rat: Twelve rats received maximum total doses of 1 g/kg bw ethylene oxide in arachis oil by s.c. injection (dosing schedule not given). The period of treatment was 94 days. The animals were observed for lifetime; no local sarcomas were observed (Walpole, 1958).

(c) Other experimental systems

Mouse: In a study not designed to test the carcinogenicity of ethylene oxide, 86 female Swiss-Webster mice, germ-free and inbred, were exposed to ethylene oxide-treated ground-corncob bedding for 150 days and then to untreated bedding for lifespan (maximal, 900 days); 63 mice developed tumours at various sites. No tumours were reported in 83 female mice, 100-600 days old, which were not exposed to treated bedding (Reyniers et al., 1964) [This observation does not allow an evaluation of the carcinogenicity of ethylene oxide].

3.2 Other relevant biological data

(a) Experimental systems

The LD_{50}'s of ethylene oxide administered intragastrically as an aqueous solution to rats and guinea-pigs are 0.33 and 0.27 g/kg bw, respectively (Smyth et al., 1941). The oral LD_{50}, when administered as a solution in olive oil to rats, is 0.2 g/kg bw (Hollingsworth et al., 1956).

In rats exposed to 15 g/m³ (8000 ppm) for 4 hours, the mortality was 6/6 (Weil et al., 1963). The LC_{50}'s were 2.6 g/m³ (1460 ppm) in rats and 1.5 g/m³ (835 ppm) in mice following 4-hour exposures (Jacobson et al., 1956). When animals were subjected to repeated 7-hour exposures of ethylene oxide vapour on 5 days per week for 6 or 7 months, guinea-pigs, rabbits and monkeys tolerated 200 mg/m³ (113 ppm), and mice and rats tolerated 90 mg/m³ (49 ppm) without adverse effects (Hollingsworth et al., 1956); while, in a similar experiment, dogs, mice and rats tolerated 183 mg/m³ (100 ppm) (Jacobson et al., 1956).

Oral administration to rats of 15 doses of 0.1 g/kg bw ethylene oxide for 21 days caused marked loss of body weight, gastric irritation and slight liver damage; no injury resulted from 22 doses of 0.03 g/kg bw over 30 days (Hollingsworth et al., 1956).

This compound has anaesthetic properties (Hollingsworth et al., 1956); and toxic doses in monkeys, rabbits and rats cause muscular atrophy of the hind-limbs (Hollingsworth et al., 1956; Jacobson et al., 1956).

Dose-related eye irritation was observed in rabbits with concentrations of over 1.8 g/m³ (1000 ppm) (McDonald et al., 1973). Exposure to high concentrations of ethylene oxide vapour caused reversible, slight fatty degeneration of the liver. Mice and rats exposed to concentrations of 0.36-1.5 g/m³ (200-850 ppm) for 7 hours a day on 5 days per week died from oedema and secondary respiratory disease (Hollingsworth et al., 1956). Ethylene oxide is 2 or 3 times as toxic as propylene oxide (Jacobson et al., 1956).

After exposure of mice to a mixture of [1,2-³H]-ethylene oxide vapour in air for 75 minutes, 90-95% of the radioactivity was eliminated in 24 hours. The highest concentrations of residual radioactivity were found in protein fractions of the spleen; smaller amounts occurred in the liver, kidney, lung and testis (Ehrenberg et al., 1974).

Ethylene oxide reacts with DNA, primarily at the N-7 position of guanosine, to form *N*-7-hydroxy-ethylguanine (Brookes & Lawley, 1961; Ehrenberg et al., 1974).

Treatment with a 9.55 mM ethanol solution of ethylene oxide for one hour at 25°C produced reverse mutations in *Salmonella typhimurium* strain TA1535 (Rannug et al., 1976). Reverse mutations were also produced in the adenine-requiring mutant strain 38701 of *Neurospora crassa* by treatment with a 0.025 M aqueous solution for 15 minutes (Kølmark & Westergaard, 1953). Ethylene oxide has induced recessive lethals (Bird, 1952; Rapoport, 1948a,b), translocations (Nakao & Auerbach, 1961; Watson, 1966) and minute mutations (Fahmy & Fahmy, 1970) in *Drosophila melanogaster*.

Exposure of male Long-Evans rats for 4 hours to 1.83 g/m^3 (1000 ppm) ethylene oxide produced dominant lethal mutations; chromosome aberrations were observed in bone-marrow cells of male Long-Evans rats exposed to 0.45 g/m^3 (250 ppm) ethylene oxide for 7 hours per day for 3 days (Embree & Hine, 1975).

(b) Man

Systemic poisoning due to exposure to ethylene oxide is rare, but 3 cases have been reported in which headache, vomiting, dyspnoea, diarrhoea and lymphocytosis occurred (Hine & Rowe, 1963). Skin burns occurred in workers in prolonged contact with a 1% solution of ethylene oxide in water (Sexton & Henson, 1949); one case of corneal burns was reported by McLaughlin (1946). Workers have developed severe skin irritation from wearing rubber gloves which had absorbed ethylene oxide; redness, oedema, blisters and ulceration were observed (Royce & Moore, 1955).

3.3 Observations in man

No data were available to the Working Group.

4. Comments on Data Reported and Evaluation

4.1 Animal data

Ethylene oxide has been tested in mice by skin application and in rats by subcutaneous injection. Although no carcinogenic effect was observed, the data do not allow an evaluation.

4.2 Human data

No case reports or epidemiological studies were available to the Working Group.

5. References

Adler, N. (1965) Residual ethylene oxide and ethylene glycol in ethylene oxide sterilized pharmaceuticals. J. pharm. Sci., 54, 735-742

Ben-Yehoshua, S. & Krinsky, P. (1968) Gas chromatography of ethylene oxide and its toxic residues. J. Gas Chromat., 6, 350-351

Berck, B. (1965) Determination of fumigant gases by gas chromatography. J. agric. Fd Chem., 13, 373-377

Binder, H. & Lindner, W. (1972) Determination of ethylene oxide in the smoke of treated and untreated cigarettes. Fachliche Mitt. Oesterr. Tabakregie 13, 215-220

Bird, M.J. (1952) Chemical production of mutations in *Drosophila*: comparison of techniques. J. Genet., 50, 480-485

Brookes, P. & Lawley, P.D. (1961) The alkylation of guanosine and guanylic acid. J. chem. Soc., 3923-3928

Brown, D.I. (1970) Determination of ethylene oxide and ethylene chlorohydrin in plastic and rubber surgical equipment sterilized with ethylene oxide. J. Ass. off. analyt. Chem., 53, 263-267

Buquet, A. & Manchon, P. (1970) Recherche et dosage des résidus et dérivés, dans un pain conservé à l'aide d'oxyde d'éthylène. Chim. analyt. (Paris) 52, 978-983

Critchfield, F.E. & Johnson, J.B. (1957) Colorimetric determination of ethylene oxide by conversion to formaldehyde. Analyt. Chem., 29, 797-800

Ehrenberg, L., Hiesche, K.D., Osterman-Golkar, S. & Wennberg, I. (1974) Evaluation of genetic risks of alkylating agents: tissue doses in the mouse from air contaminated with ethylene oxide. Mutation Res., 24, 83-103

Embree, J.W. & Hine, C.H. (1975) Mutagenicity of ethylene oxide. Toxicol. appl. Pharmacol., 33, 172-173

Fahmy, O.G. & Fahmy, M.J. (1970) Gene elimination in carcinogenesis: re-interpretation of the somatic mutation theory. Cancer Res., 30, 195-205

FAO/WHO (1972) 1971 Evaluations of Some Pesticide Residues in Food. Report of the 1971 Joint Meeting of the FAO Working Party of Experts on Pesticide Residues and the WHO Expert Committee on Pesticide Residues. WHO Pest. Res. Series, No. 1, pp. 280-288

Fishbein, L. (1969) Degradation and residues of alkylating agents. Ann. N.Y. Acad. Sci., 163, 869-894

Gage, J.C. (1957) The determination of ethylene oxide in the atmosphere. Analyst, 82, 587-589

Gunther, D.A. (1965) Determination of adsorbed ethylene and propylene oxides by distillation and titration. Analyt. Chem., 37, 1172-1173

Hawley, G.G., ed. (1971) The Condensed Chemical Dictionary, New York, Van Nostrand-Reinhold, p. 367

Heuser, S.G. & Scudamore, K.A. (1968) Fumigant residues in wheat and flour: solvent extraction and gas-chromatographic determination of free methyl bromide and ethylene oxide. Analyst, 93, 252-258

Heuser, S.G. & Scudamore, K.A. (1969) Determination of fumigant residues in cereals and other foodstuffs: a multi-detection scheme for gas chromatography of solvent extracts. J. Sci. Fd Agric., 20, 566-572

Hine, C.H. & Rowe, V.K. (1963) Ethylene oxide. In: Patty, F.A., ed. Industrial Hygiene and Toxicology, 2nd ed., Vol. 2, New York, Interscience, pp. 1626-1634

Hollingsworth, R.L. & Waling, B.F. (1955) Determination of ethylene oxide in air. Experience in the use of Lubatti's method. Amer. industr. Hyg. Ass. Quart., 16, 52-54

Hollingsworth, R.L., Rowe, V.K., Oyen, F., McCollister, D.D. & Spencer, H.C. (1956) Toxicity of ethylene oxide determined on experimental animals. Arch. industr. Hlth, 13, 217-227

Jacobson, K.H., Hackley, E.B. & Feinsilver, L. (1956) The toxicity of inhaled ethylene oxide and propylene oxide vapours. Arch. industr. Hlth, 13, 237-244

Kaliberdo, L.M. & Vaabel, A.S. (1967) Quantitative determination of lower olefin oxides in their mixture with aldehydes by gas-liquid chromatography. Zh. analyt. Khim., 22, 1590-1592

Kølmark, G. & Westergaard, M. (1953) Further studies on chemically induced reversions at the adenine locus of Neurospora. Hereditas, 39, 209-224

Kulkarni, R.K., Bartak, D., Ousterhout, D.K. & Leonard, F. (1968) Determination of residual ethylene oxide in catheters by gas-liquid chromatography. J. Biomed. Mater. Res., 2, 165-171

Lubatti, O.F. (1944) Determination of fumigants. XIV. Residual ethylene oxide in wheat. J. Soc. chem. industr. Transact. (Lond.), 63, 133-139

Manchon, P. & Buquet, A. (1970) Determination et dosage de l'oxyde d'éthylène (oxirane) et de ses dérivés dans le pain traité par ce fumigant. Fd Cosmet. Toxicol., 8, 9-15

McDonald, T.O., Kasten, K., Hervey, R., Gregg, S., Borgmann, A.R. & Murchison, T. (1973) Acute ocular toxicity of ethylene oxide, ethylene glycol and ethylene chlorohydrin. Bull. parent. Drug Ass., 27, 153-164

McLaughlin, R.S. (1946) Chemical burns of the human cornea. Amer. J. Ophthal., 29, 1355-1362

Muramatsu, M., Obi, Y., Shimada, Y., Takahashi, K. & Nishida, K. (1968) Ethylene oxide in cigarette smoke. Rep. centr. Res. Lab. Jap. Monop. Manuf., 110, 217-222

Nakao, Y. & Auerbach, C. (1961) Test of a possible correlation between cross-linking and chromosome breaking abilities of chemical mutagens. Z. Vererbungsl., 92, 457-461

Pozzoli, L., Bobbio, G. & Armeli, G. (1968) Spectrophotometric determination of ethylene and propylene oxides and ethyl and butyl alcohols in air. Lav. umano, 20, 409-417

Preussmann, R., Schneider, H. & Epple, F. (1969) Untersuchungen zum Nachweis alkylierender Agentien. II. Der Nachweis verschiedener Klassen alkylierender Agentien mit einder Modifikation der Farbreaktion mit 4-(4'-Nitrobenzyl)pyridin (NBP). Arzneimittelforsch., 19, 1059-1073

Ragelis, E.P., Fisher, B.S. & Klimeck, B.A. (1966) Note on determination of chlorohydrins in foods fumigated with ethylene oxide and with propylene oxide. J. Ass. off. analyt. Chem., 49, 963-965

Rannug, U., Göthe, R. & Wachtmeister, C.A. (1976) The mutagenicity of chloroethylene oxide, chloroacetaldehyde, 2-chloroethanol and chloroacetic acid, conceivable metabolites of vinyl chloride. Chem.-biol. Interact. (in press)

Rapoport, I.A. (1948a) Alkylation of gene molecule. Dokl. Akad. Nauk SSR, 59, 1183-1186

Rapoport, I.A. (1948b) Action of ethylene oxide, glycidol and glycols on gene mutation. Dokl. Akad. Nauk SSR, 60, 469-472

Redaelli, G., Marazza, V. & Reina, G. (1967) Determination and persistence of ethylene oxide in meat, fish, and bone meals after sterilization. Clin. Vet., 90, 67-71

Reyniers, J.A., Sacksteder, M.R. & Ashburn, L.L. (1964) Multiple tumors in female germfree inbred albino mice exposed to bedding treated with ethylene oxide. J. nat. Cancer Inst., 32, 1045-1057

Royce, A. & Moore, W.K.S. (1955) Occupational dermatitis caused by ethylene oxide. Brit. J. industr. Med., 12, 169-171

Sexton, R.J. & Henson, E.V. (1949) Dermatological injuries by ethylene oxide. J. industr. Hyg. Toxicol., 31, 297-300

Smyth, H.F., Jr, Seaton, J. & Fischer, L. (1941) Single dose toxicity of some glycols and derivatives. J. industr. Hyg. Toxicol., 23, 259-268

Stecher, P.G., ed. (1968) The Merck Index, 8th ed., Rahway, NJ, Merck & Co., p. 435

Swan, J.D. (1954) Determination of epoxides with sodium sulfite. Analyt. Chem., 26, 878-880

US Code of Federal Regulations (1974) Protection of Environment, Title 40, part 180.151, Washington DC, US Government Printing Office, p. 259

US Environmental Protection Agency (1973) EPA Compendium of Registered Pesticides, Vol. II, Fungicides and Nematicides, Washington DC, US Government Printing Office, p. E-05-00.01

US International Trade Commission (1975) Synthetic Organic Chemicals, US Production and Sales, 1973, ITC Publication 728, Washington DC, US Government Printing Office, p. 205

US Tariff Commission (1922) Census of Dyes and Other Synthetic Organic Chemicals, 1921, Tariff Information Series No. 26, Washington DC, US Government Printing Office, p. 150

Van Duuren, B.L., Orris, L. & Nelson, N. (1965) Carcinogenicity of epoxides, lactones and peroxy compounds. II. J. nat. Cancer Inst., 35, 707-717

Walpole, A.L. (1958) Carcinogenic action of alkylating agents. Ann. N.Y. Acad. Sci., 68, 750-761

Watson, W.A.F. (1966) Further evidence of an essential difference between the genetical effects of mono- and bifunctional alkylating agents. Mutation Res., 3, 455-457

Weil, C.S., Condra, N., Haun, C. & Striegel, J.A. (1963) Experimental carcinogenicity and acute toxicity of representative epoxides. Amer. industr. Hyg. Ass. J., 24, 305-325

Wesley, F., Rourke, B. & Darbishire, O. (1965) The formation of persistent toxic chlorohydrins in foodstuffs by fumigation with ethylene oxide and with propylene oxide. J. Fd Sci., 30, 1037-1042

Winell, M.A. (1975) An international comparison of hygienic standards for chemicals in the work environment. Ambio, 4, 34-36

FUSARENON-X*

1. Chemical and Physical Data

1.1 Synonyms and trade names

Chem. Abstr. Reg. Serial No.: 23255-69-8

Chem. Abstr. Name: 4-Acetyloxy-12,13-epoxy-3,7,15-trihydroxy-(3α,4β,7β)-trichothec-9-en-8-one

Fusarenon; fusarenone X; 3,7,15-trihydroxy-4-acetoxy-8-oxo-12,13-epoxy-Δ^9-trichothecene; 3,7,15-trihydroxyscirp-4-acetoxy-9-en-8-one; nivalenol-4-O-acetate

1.2 Chemical formula and molecular weight

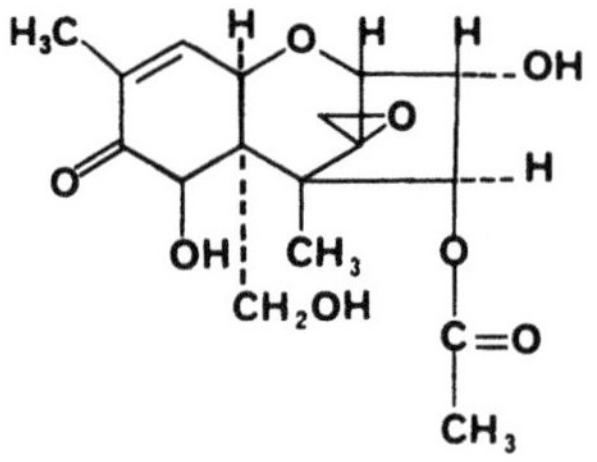

$C_{17}H_{22}O_8$ Mol. wt: 354

1.3 Chemical and physical properties

(a) Description: Transparent crystals

(b) Melting-point: 91-92°C

(c) Optical rotation: $[\alpha]_D^{25}$ +58° (1% in methanol); $[\alpha]_D^{24}$ +56°C (in ethanol)

(d) Spectroscopy data: λ_{max} 220 nm (in methanol); infra-red carbonyl band at 1680 cm^{-1}

---

*Considered by the Working Group, February 1976

(e) Solubility: Soluble in water, ethyl acetate, ethanol, methanol and chloroform; insoluble in n-hexane and n-pentane.

(f) Reactivity: Susceptible to hydrolysis to form nivalenol

1.4 Technical products and impurities

No data were available to the Working Group.

2. Production, Use, Occurrence and Analysis

2.1 Production and use

Fusarenon-X is not produced commercially.

2.2 Occurrence

Fusarenon-X is formed by fungi such as *Fusarium nivale*, *F. episphaeria*, *F. oxysporum* and *Gibberella zeae* (Smalley & Strong, 1974; Ueno *et al.*, 1972a, 1973).

Strains such as *F. nivale* and *G. zeae* have occasionally been isolated from scabbed wheat grains in Japan (Tsunoda, 1970; Ueno *et al.*, 1972b), and 20% of domestic wheat and barley samples were found to be contaminated by such fungi (Tsuruta, 1974).

2.3 Analysis

Analytical methods employing thin-layer chromatography (limits of detection, 0.1-0.2 µg) (Ueno *et al.*, 1973) and gas chromatography (Saito & Ohtsubo, 1974) have been described.

3. Biological Data Relevant to the Evaluation of Carcinogenic Risk to Man

3.1 Carcinogenicity and related studies in animals

(a) Oral administration

Rat: A group of 20 male 8-week old Donryu rats was given 0.4 mg/kg bw fusarenon-X weekly by oral intubation. Twelve rats survived 50 weeks, and 1 developed a hepatoma. No tumours occurred in 10 male controls during the experimental period of over 400 days (Saito & Ohtsubo, 1974).

(b) Subcutaneous and/or intramuscular administration

Mouse: Two groups of 16 and 18 8-week old male DDD mice received 10 or 20 weekly s.c. injections of 2.5 mg/kg bw fusarenon-X and were observed for up to 400 days. One case of leukaemia was observed. No tumours occurred in 11 control mice during the experimental period of over 400 days (Saito & Ohtsubo, 1974).

Rat: Eighteen 8-week old male Donryu rats were given weekly s.c. injections of 0.4 mg/kg bw fusarenon-X for 22 weeks; most of the rats survived more than 1 year, and 1 developed a lung adenoma. No tumours were seen in 10 controls (Saito & Ohtsubo, 1974).

3.2 Other relevant biological data

(a) Experimental systems

The i.p. LD_{50} of fusarenon-X in male and female mice was 3.4 mg/kg bw; the s.c. LD_{50} in newborn mice was 0.1 mg/kg bw; the oral LD_{50}'s in male and female Wistar rats were 4.4 and 4.0 mg/kg bw, respectively; the i.p. LD_{50} in guinea-pigs was about 0.5 mg/kg bw (Ueno, 1971; Ueno et al., 1971a).

Rats and mice administered fusarenon-X had cytotoxic damage in the mucosa of the small intestine, in the germ centres of the lymph follicles and in the spleen, lymph nodes, thymus and bone marrow. Fusarenon-X, as other trichothecene compounds, causes severe irritation of the skin (Ueno, 1971; Ueno et al., 1970, 1971b).

Following its i.p. injection in mice, most of a dose of ^{3}H-fusarenon-X was rapidly excreted in the urine; almost no radioactivity remained in the tissues after 3 hours. Fusarenon-X was shown to be metabolized into uncharacterized polar compounds (Ueno et al., 1971a).

(c) Man

Splashing of a crude solution caused irritating dermatitis of the hands and face in laboratory workers (Saito & Ohtsubo, 1974).

3.3 Observations in man

No data were available to the Working Group.

4. Comments on Data Reported and Evaluation

4.1 Animal data

Fusarenon-X was inadequately tested in mice and rats. No assessment of its carcinogenicity can be made.

4.2 Human data

No case reports or epidemiological studies were available to the Working Group.

5. References

Saito, M. & Ohtsubo, K. (1974) Trichothecene toxins of *Fusarium* species. In: Purchase, I.F.H., ed., Mycotoxins, Amsterdam, Elsevier, pp. 263-289

Smalley, E.B. & Strong, F.M. (1974) Toxic trichothecenes. In: Purchase, I.F.H., ed., Mycotoxins, Amsterdam, Elsevier, pp. 199-228

Tsunoda, H. (1970) Micro-organisms which deteriorate stored cereals and grains. In: Herzberg, M., ed., Proceedings of the 1st US-Japan Conference on Toxic Micro-organisms, Washington DC, US Department of the Interior, pp. 143-162

Tsuruta, A. (1974) Micro-organisms infection of domestic cereals. I. Parasitic fungi on wheat and barley. Fd Res. Inst. (Tokyo), 29, 16-20

Ueno, Y. (1971) Toxicological and biological properties of fusarenon-X, a cytotoxic mycotoxin of *Fusarium nivale* Fn 2B. In: Purchase, I.F.H., ed., Mycotoxins in Human Health, London, Macmillan, pp. 163-178

Ueno, Y., Ishikawa, Y., Amakai, K., Nakajima, M., Saito, M., Enomoto, M. & Ohtsubo, K. (1970) Comparative study on skin-necrotizing effect of scirpene metabolites of *Fusaria*. Jap. J. exp. Med., 40, 33-38

Ueno, Y., Ueno, I., Iitoi, Y., Tsunoda, H., Enomoto, M. & Ohtsubo, K. (1971a) Toxicological approaches to the metabolites of *Fusaria*. III. Acute toxicity of fusarenon-X. Jap. J. exp. Med., 41, 521-539

Ueno, Y., Ishikawa, Y., Nakajima, M., Sakai, K., Ishii, K., Tsunoda, H., Saito, M., Enomoto, M., Ohtsubo, K. & Umeda, M. (1971b) Toxicological approaches to the metabolites of *Fusaria*. I. Screening of toxic strains. Jap. J. exp. Med., 41, 257-272

Ueno, Y., Sato, N., Ishii, K., Sakai, K. & Enomoto, M. (1972a) Toxicological approaches to the metabolites of *Fusaria*. V. Neosolaniol, T-2 toxin and butenolide, toxic metabolites of *Fusarium sporotrichioides* NRRL 3510 and *Fusarium poae* 3287. Jap. J. exp. Med., 42, 461-472

Ueno, Y., Ishii, K., Sakai, K., Kanaeda, S., Tsunoda, H., Tanaka, T. & Enomoto, M. (1972b) Toxicological approaches to the metabolites of *Fusaria*. IV. Microbial survey on 'bean-hulls poisoning of horses' with the isolation of toxic trichothecenes, neosolaniol and T-2 toxin of *Fusarium solani* M-1-1. Jap. J. exp. Med., 42, 187-203

Ueno, Y., Sato, N., Ishii, K., Sakai, K., Tsunoda, H. & Enomoto, M. (1973) Biological and chemical detection of trichothecene mycotoxins of *Fusarium* species. Appl. Microbiol., 25, 699-704

GLYCIDALDEHYDE*

1. Chemical and Physical Data

1.1 Synonyms and trade names

Chem. Abstr. Reg. Serial No.: 765-34-4

Chem. Abstr. Name: Oxirane-carboxaldehyde

Epihydrinaldehyde; epihydrine aldehyde; 2,3-epoxypropanal; 2,3-epoxy-1-propanal; 2,3-epoxypropionaldehyde; glycidal; glycidyl aldehyde

1.2 Chemical formula and molecular weight

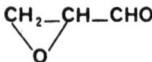

$C_3H_4O_2$ Mol. wt: 72.1

1.3 Chemical and physical properties

(a) Description: Colourless liquid

(b) Boiling-point: 112-113°C at 760 mm; 53°C at 101 mm

(c) Density: d_4^{20} 1.1403

(d) Refractive index: n_D^{22} 1.4225; n_D^{20} 1.4198

(e) Spectroscopy data: Infra-red carbonyl band at 1730 cm^{-1} and epoxide band at 1228 cm^{-1}

(f) Solubility: Miscible with water and all common solvents; immiscible with petroleum ether

---

*Considered by the Working Group, February 1976. This compound should be clearly distinguished from glyceraldehyde ($CH_2OH.CHOH.CHO$) which does not contain the epoxy group.

(g) Stability: Undiluted glycidaldehyde is stable at room temperature, but a 30% aqueous solution lost 94% of the epoxide after 2 months at room temperature.

(h) Reactivity: The aldehyde and epoxide groups are both reactive.

1.4 Technical products and impurities

No data were available to the Working Group.

2. Production, Use, Occurrence and Analysis

For important background information on this section, see preamble, p. 19.

2.1 Production and use

Acrolein can be converted to glycidaldehyde by the action of hydrogen peroxide (at pH 8) or sodium hypochlorite (Guest et al., 1963).

No evidence was found that glycidaldehyde has ever been produced or used commercially in the US; however, in the UK, it has been used as a cross-linking agent for the finishing of wool, for the oil tanning ('chamoising') and fat-liquoring of leather and surgical sutures and for protein insolubilization (Hine & Rowe, 1963).

Glycidaldehyde has been tested as a vapour-phase disinfectant (Dawson, 1962). It inactivates foot-and-mouth virus and can be used in the preparation of an immune serum for the protection of animals against that disease (McKerche & Giordano, 1967).

A process for making glycerine from acrolein via glycidaldehyde has been suggested (Guest et al., 1963).

2.2 Occurrence

Glycidaldehyde occurs in sunflower oil, and its concentration increases with that of peroxides during storage, causing deterioration of the flavour. To maintain a high quality of the oil, peroxides should not exceed 0.25% and glycidaldehyde not more than 0.46 mg/ml (Romysh & Dubenetskaya, 1967). Glycidaldehyde has been detected in rancid samples of commercial lard (Woller & Nagy, 1968).

2.3 Analysis

Glycidaldehyde has been determined in air by use of a gas scrubber containing hydrochloric acid in saturated aqueous magnesium chloride solution, followed by titration with sodium hydroxide (Dawson, 1962). Its determination in fats may be made colorimetrically (Fomin et al., 1963). See also 'General Remarks on the Substances Considered', p. 29.

3. Biological Data Relevant to the Evaluation of Carcinogenic Risk to Man

3.1 Carcinogenicity and related studies in animals

(a) Skin application

Mouse: Applications of a 3% solution of glycidaldehyde in benzene on the clipped dorsal skin of 8-week old female ICR/Ha Swiss mice thrice weekly for life resulted in the development of skin tumours in 16/30 animals; 8 had papillomas and 8 had carcinomas (Van Duuren et al., 1965).

A group of 41 8-week old female ICR/Ha Swiss mice received thrice weekly applications on the dorsal skin of 10 mg glycidaldehyde as a 10% solution in acetone. Skin papillomas developed in 6/41 mice; 3 of these had squamous-cell carcinomas of the skin after 308 days. The median survival time was longer than 526 days. No skin tumours were seen in 300 acetone-treated controls (Van Duuren et al., 1967a) [$P<0.01$].

(b) Subcutaneous and/or intramuscular administration

Mouse: Two groups of 30 and 50 8-week old female ICR/Ha Swiss mice were given weekly s.c. injections of 3.3 or 0.1 mg glycidaldehyde in 0.05 ml tricaprylin. Local sarcomas and squamous-cell carcinomas were produced in 5/30 and 3/50 mice at the two doses, respectively. No local tumours developed in 110 tricaprylin-injected controls (Van Duuren et al., 1966) [$P<0.01$].

Rat: Two groups of 20 and 50 6-week old female Sprague-Dawley rats received weekly s.c. injections of 33 or 1 mg glycidaldehyde in 0.1 ml tricaprylin. Local sarcomas occurred in 5/20 and 1/50 rats at the two dose levels, respectively (maximum duration of tests, 539 and 558 days).

Tricaprylin-injected and untreated controls developed no local tumours (maximum duration of tests, 554 and 565 days) (Van Duuren et al., 1966, 1967b).

3.2 Other relevant biological data

(a) Experimental systems

The LD_{50} of intragastrically administered glycidaldehyde in rats was 230 mg/kg bw; the LC_{50} in rats for a 9-32-hour exposure by inhalation was 735 mg/m^3 (250 ppm). In rabbits, the percutaneous LD_{50} of glycidaldehyde was 250 mg/kg bw; none of 3 animals died after a skin application of 40 mg/kg bw, although severe local injury occurred.

Sixty 4-hour exposures to 29 mg/m^3 (10 ppm) glycidaldehyde vapour in air had no effect on rats; concentrations of 60 mg/m^3 (20 ppm) and of 118 mg/m^3 (40 ppm) resulted in retardations in body-weight gain, several deaths and some effects on the haematopoietic system. Exposure to 235 mg/m^3 (80 ppm) caused the death of 8/10 rats before the 5th exposure, with focal necrosis of liver and kidney (Hine et al., 1961).

Glycidaldehyde is irritating to surface tissues and mucous membranes. Repeated i.v. injections into rabbits lowered the leucocyte count and the proportion of polymorphonuclear cells; the number of nucleated marrow cells was significantly decreased in rats exposed chronically to the vapour (Hine et al., 1961; Kodama et al., 1961).

Exposure of bacteriophage T4 to a 300-fold dilution of glycidaldehyde for 30 minutes at 37°C induced mutations in the rII region of the phage by producing base-pair transitions (primarily A-T to G-C), frameshift mutations and some deletions (Corbett et al., 1970).

Glycidaldehyde has also produced base-pair mutations in two strains of *Salmonella typhimurium* (TA1535 and TA1000) (McCann et al., 1975). A 1% solution in ethanol induced reverse base-pair mutations in *Saccharomyces cerevisiae* strain S211; a 2-4% solution induced petites cytoplasmic mutations in strain N123 of the same organism (Izard, 1973).

(b) Man

Glycidaldehyde produces marked skin irritation with slow healing, following by pigmentation. According to Hine & Rowe (1963), several cases of skin sensitization have occurred. They suggested that an atmospheric concentration of 2.94 mg/m^3 (1 ppm) be set as a 'permissible exposure', on the basis of comfort (avoidance of skin and nasal irritation) and potential haemopoietic effects.

3.3 Observations in man

No data were available to the Working Group.

4. Comments on Data Reported and Evaluation[1]

4.1 Animal data

Glycidaldehyde is carcinogenic in mice by skin application and by subcutaneous injection and in rats by subcutaneous injection. It produced malignant tumours at the site of application in both species.

4.2 Human data

No case reports or epidemiological studies were available to the Working Group.

---

[1]See also the section 'Animal Data in Relation to the Evaluation of Risk to Man' in the introduction to this volume, p. 17.

5. References

Corbett, T.H., Heidelberger, C. & Dove, W.F. (1970) Determination of the mutagenic activity to bacteriophage T4 of carcinogenic and noncarcinogenic compounds. *Molec. Pharmacol.*, 6, 667-679

Dawson, F.W. (1962) Glycidaldehyde vapor as a disinfectant. *Amer. J. Hyg.*, 76, 209-215

Fomin, A.A., Fedorov, N.A. & Kasatkin, I.N. (1963) Quantitative determination of fatty acids using distributive paper chromatography. *Vop. Med. Khim.*, 9, 76-79

Guest, H.F., Kiff, B.W. & Stansbury, H.A., Jr (1963) *Acrolein and derivatives*. In: Kirk, R.E. & Othmer, D.F., eds, *Encyclopedia of Chemical Technology*, 2nd ed., Vol. 1, New York, John Wiley and Sons, pp. 261-262

Hine, C.H. & Rowe, V.K. (1963) *Glycidaldehyde*. In: Patty, F.A., ed., *Industrial Hygiene and Toxicology*, 2nd ed., Vol. 2, New York, Interscience, pp. 1635-1637

Hine, C.H., Guzman, R.J., Dunlap, M.K., Lima, R. & Loquvam, G.S. (1961) Studies on the toxicity of glycidaldehyde. *Arch. environm. Hlth*, 2, 23-30

Izard, M.C. (1973) Recherches sur les effets mutagènes de l'acroléine et de ses deux époxydes: le glycidol et le glycidal, sur *Saccharomyces cerevisiae*. *C.R. Acad. Sci. (Paris)*, 276, 3037-3041

Kodama, J.K., Guzman, R.J., Dunlap, M.K., Loquvam, G.S., Lima, R. & Hine, C.H. (1961) Some effects of epoxy compounds on the blood. *Arch. environm. Hlth*, 2, 50-61

McCann, J., Choi, E., Yamasaki, E. & Ames, B.N. (1975) Detection of carcinogens as mutagens in the *Salmonella*/microsome test. Assay of 300 chemicals. *Proc. nat. Acad. Sci. (Wash.)*, 72, 5135-5139

McKercher, P.D. & Giordano, A.R. (1967) Immune response of steers inoculated with chemically-treated foot-and-mouth disease virus preparations previously studied in swine. *Arch. ges. Virusforsch.*, 20, 190-197

Romysh, L.F. & Dubenetskaya, M.M. (1967) Standards for oxidative spoilage of sunflower oil. *Vop. Pitan.*, 26, 82-87

Van Duuren, B.L., Orris, L. & Nelson, N. (1965) Carcinogenicity of epoxides, lactones and peroxy compounds. II. *J. nat. Cancer Inst.*, 35, 707-717

Van Duuren, B.L., Langseth, L., Orris, L., Teebor, G., Nelson, N. & Kuschner, M. (1966) Carcinogenicity of epoxides, lactones and peroxy compounds. IV. Tumor response in epithelial and connective tissue in mice and rats. J. nat. Cancer Inst., 37, 825-834

Van Duuren, B.L., Langseth, L., Goldschmidt, B.M. & Orris, L. (1967a) Carcinogenicity of epoxides, lactones and peroxy compounds. VI. Structure and carcinogenic activity. J. nat. Cancer Inst., 39, 1217-1228

Van Duuren, B.L., Langseth, L., Orris, L., Baden, M. & Kuschner, M. (1967b) Carcinogenicity of epoxides, lactones and peroxy compounds. V. Subcutaneous injection in rats. J. nat. Cancer Inst., 39, 1213-1216

Woller, R. & Nagy, M. (1968) Changes in lard during storage. I. Fleischwirtschaft, 48, 810-812

GLYCIDYL OLEATE*

1. Chemical and Physical Data

1.1 Synonyms and trade names

Chem. Abstr. Reg. Serial No.: 5431-33-4

Chem. Abstr. Name: Oxiranylmethyl ester of 9-octadecenoic acid

2,3-Epoxy-1-propanol oleate; 2,3-epoxypropyl ester of oleic acid; 2,3-epoxypropyl oleate; glycidol oleate; glycidyl octadecenoate; oleic acid glycidyl ester

1.2 Chemical formula and molecular weight

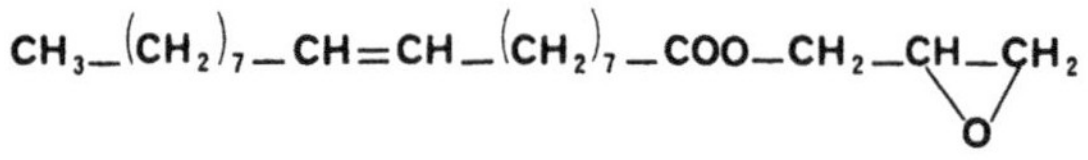

$$CH_3-(CH_2)_7-CH=CH-(CH_2)_7-COO-CH_2-CH-CH_2$$
$$\diagdown O \diagup$$

$C_{21}H_{38}O_3$ Mol. wt: 338.5

1.3 Chemical and physical properties

(a) Description: Colourless oil

(b) Boiling-point: 185-190°C at 1 mm

(c) Melting-point: -0.5°C

(d) Stability: Susceptible to autoxidation and to hydrolysis

(e) Reactivity: Both the epoxide and the double bond are reactive.

1.4 Technical products and impurities

No data were available to the Working Group.

---

*Considered by the Working Group, February 1976

2. Production, Use, Occurrence and Analysis

For important background information on this section, see preamble, p. 19.

2.1 Production and use

Glycidyl oleate can be prepared by treating potassium oleate with epichlorohydrin in the presence of benzyltrimethylammonium chloride (Carreau, 1970).

Although patents have been issued on the use of glycidyl oleate as an intermediate for the corresponding dihydroxy ester (2,3-dihydroxypropyl oleate) and for the production of modified proteins recommended for use in the treatment of damaged hair, no indication was found that it has been used for such purposes.

2.2 Occurrence

No data were available to the Working Group.

2.3 Analysis

See section 'General Remarks on the Substances Considered', p. 29.

3. Biological Data Relevant to the Evaluation of Carcinogenic Risk to Man

3.1 Carcinogenicity and related studies in animals

Subcutaneous and/or intramuscular administration

Mouse: Of 15 8-week old female BALB/c mice given twice weekly s.c. injections of 0.25 mg/animal glycidyl oleate in 0.1 ml tricaprylin for 52 week, 10 survived 9 or more months, and 5 developed local sarcomas after 10-11 months. Of 7 controls injected with tricaprylin alone and surviving 9 or more months, 1 developed a local sarcoma after 13 months; 5 survived longer than 18 months (Swern *et al.*, 1970) [P>0.05].

3.2 Other relevant biological data

Experimental systems

The oral LD_{50} of glycidyl oleate in rats was 3.5 ml/kg bw; the percutaneous LD_{50} in rabbits was 8.0 ml/kg bw. Rats survived an 8-hour exposure to an atmosphere saturated with glycidyl oleate vapour (Weil et al., 1963).

Glycidyl oleate was only weakly irritating to surface and mucous membranes. Two of three guinea-pigs that were tested by an intra-cutaneous injection became sensitized to this substance (Weil et al., 1963).

3.3 Observations in man

No data were available to the Working Group.

4. Comments on Data Reported and Evaluation

4.1 Animal data

Glycidyl oleate has been tested in a limited study in mice in which subcutaneous injection produced a low incidence of local sarcomas. This result is insufficient for evaluation.

4.2 Human data

No case reports or epidemiological studies were available to the Working Group.

5. References

Carreau, J.P. (1970) Syntheses of triglycerides with three different fatty acids. I. Preparation of glycidol esters. Bull. Soc. chim. Fr., 11, 4104-4106

Swern, D., Wieder, R., McDonough, M., Meranze, D.R. & Shimkin, M.B. (1970) Investigation of fatty acids and derivatives for carcinogenic activity. Cancer Res., 30, 1037-1046

Weil, C.S., Condra, N., Haun, C. & Striegel, J.A. (1963) Experimental carcinogenicity and acute toxicity of representative epoxides. Amer. industr. Hyg. Ass. J., 24, 304-325

GLYCIDYL STEARATE*

1. Chemical and Physical Data

1.1 Synonyms and trade names

Chem. Abstr. Reg. Serial No.: 7460-84-6

Chem. Abstr. Name: Oxiranylmethyl ester of octadecanoic acid

2,3-Epoxy-1-propanol stearate; 2,3-epoxypropyl ester of stearic acid; 2,3-epoxypropyl stearate; glycidol stearate; glycidyl octadecanoate; stearic acid glycidyl ester

1.2 Chemical formula and molecular weight

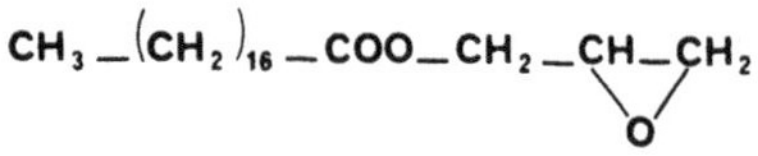

$$CH_3-(CH_2)_{16}-COO-CH_2-CH-CH_2$$
$$\diagdown O \diagup$$

$C_{21}H_{40}O_3$ Mol. wt: 340.6

1.3 Chemical and physical properties

(a) Description: Solid

(b) Melting-point: 52°C

(c) Solubility: Sparingly soluble in water

(d) Stability: Slowly hydrolysed in water

(e) Reactivity: The epoxide group is reactive.

1.4 Technical products and impurities

No data were available to the Working Group.

---

*Considered by the Working Group, February 1976

2. Production, Use, Occurrence and Analysis

For important background information on this section, see preamble, p. 19.

2.1 Production and use

Glycidyl stearate can be prepared by treating stearic acid or its salts with epichlorohydrin in the presence of a quaternary ammonium halide and an alkali metal salt (Nevin & Fletcher, 1961). It has also been made by the catalytic hydrogenation of glycidyl linoleate (Anon., 1969).

Patents have been issued on the use of glycidyl stearate as an intermediate in a number of reactions: for the corresponding dihydroxy ester (2,3-dihydroxypropyl stearate); for condensates with short-chain polyamines (e.g., diethylenetriamine), with polyethylenimine (recommended as textile softeners) or with dialkyl amines (recommended as antistatic agents for plastics); for mixed triglycerides containing three different fatty acid substituents; for polymerization to waxes; and for the production of modified proteins recommended for use in the treatment of damaged hair. However, no indication was found that the compound is used in such applications.

2.2 Occurrence

No data were available to the Working Group.

2.3 Analysis

See section 'General Remarks on the Substances Considered', p. 29.

3. Biological Data Relevant to the Evaluation of Carcinogenic Risk to Man

3.1 Carcinogenicity and related studies in animals

Subcutaneous and/or intramuscular administration

Mouse: One group of 12 female BALB/c mice and 2 groups of 16 female Swiss Webster mice (age at start not specified) were given twice weekly or weekly s.c. injections of glycidyl stearate in doses of 10 mg, 0.1 mg and 0.005 mg per injection in tricaprylin for 33 or 26 weeks (total doses 660, 2.6 and 0.13 mg/animal, respectively). At all doses, 1 animal/group developed a local sarcoma after 16-23 months. The numbers of animals surviving 15 or more months were 10, 13 and 13 in the three groups, respectively. One local sarcoma occurred among 10 BALB/c controls injected with tricaprylin alone; 5 of these survived 15 or more months. No local tumours occurred in 3 other groups of 15-29 Swiss Webster mice injected with tricaprylin alone, once or thrice weekly; only 9 of these controls survived 18 or more months (Swern et al., 1970).

In studies conducted in two different laboratories the same chemical was administered in tricaprylin by s.c. injection once weekly for 26 weeks at 2 dose levels (0.05 or 0.1 mg) to groups of 15 or 16 ICR/Ha Swiss or Swiss Webster mice (age at start not specified). One local sarcoma was observed in each test group; no local sarcomas occurred in the 46 vehicle-injected controls (Van Duuren et al., 1972).

3.2 Other relevant biological data

No data were available to the Working Group.

3.3 Observations in man

No data were available to the Working Group.

4. Comments on Data Reported and Evaluation

4.1 Animal data

Glycidyl stearate was tested in mice by subcutaneous injection; it produced no significant increase in the incidence of local tumours.

4.2 Human data

No case reports or epidemiological studies were available to the Working Group.

5. References

Anon. (1969) Hydrogenation of glycidyl ethers or esters. French Patent 1,556,501, February 7, to Ciba Ltd

Nevin, C.S. & Fletcher, J.H. (1961) Glycidyl esters of higher fatty acids. US Patent 2,992,239, July 1, to American Cyanamid Co.

Swern, D., Wieder, R., McDonough, M., Meranze, D.R. & Shimkin, M.B. (1970) Investigation of fatty acids and derivatives for carcinogenic activity. Cancer Res., 30, 1037-1046

Van Duuren, B.L., Katz, C., Shimkin, M.B., Swern, D. & Wieder, R. (1972) Replication of low-level carcinogenic activity bioassays. Cancer Res., 32, 880-881

PROPYLENE OXIDE*

1. Chemical and Physical Data

1.1 Synonyms and trade names

Chem. Abstr. Reg. Serial No.: 75-56-9

Chem. Abstr. Name: Methyloxirane

Epoxypropane; 1,2-epoxypropane; methyl ethylene oxide; methyl oxirane; propeneoxide; propene oxide; propyleneoxide; 1,2-propylene oxide

1.2 Chemical formula and molecular weight

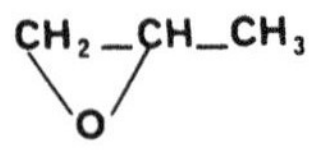

$$CH_2 - CH - CH_3$$
$$\diagdown O \diagup$$

C_3H_6O Mol. wt: 58.1

1.3 Chemical and physical properties

(a) Description: Colourless liquid

(b) Boiling-point: 35°C

(c) Density: d_4^0 0.859; d_{20}^{20} 0.831

(d) Solubility: Miscible with water (40.5% at 20°C; 59% at 25°C); miscible with common organic solvents

(e) Refractive index: n_D^{25} 1.363

(f) Reactivity: Reacts with active hydrogen compounds (e.g., alcohols, amines) and with inorganic chloride in foods to form 1-chloro-2-propanol (Ragelis *et al.*, 1966; Wesley *et al.*, 1965). Also reacts with 4-(4'-nitrobenzyl)pyridine (Preussmann *et al.*, 1969)

---

*Considered by the Working Group, February 1976

1.4 Technical products and impurities

Propylene oxide is available, in drums or tank cars, from one US producer as a product of 99.99% purity. Another producer gives the following specifications: acetic acid, 0.005%; water, 0.01%; propionaldehyde, 0.05%; boiling range, 33.0-37.0°C; and no residual odour.

2. Production, Use, Occurrence and Analysis

For important background information on this section, see preamble, p. 19.

2.1 Production and use

Propylene oxide was prepared in 1861 by Oser from 1-chloro-2-propanol and potassium hydroxide (Mark *et al.*, 1967). Until 1969, essentially all the propylene oxide produced in the US was by the chlorohydrin process (Stecher, 1968). In that year, the first US plant using a peroxidation process started production, and by mid-1973, 70% of the propylene oxide in the US was produced by the chlorohydrin process and 30% by the peroxidation process. The peroxidation process is based on the oxidation of isobutane to tertiary-butyl hydroperoxide and tertiary-butyl alcohol. The tertiary-butyl hydroperoxide, after separation, is used to oxidize propylene to propylene oxide. Ethyl benzene can be substituted for isobutane in this process.

Propylene oxide was first produced commercially in the US in 1925 (US Tariff Commission, 1926). In July 1973, there were 5 major companies, and total production in that year was 796 million kg (US International Trade Commission, 1975). In 1972, US imports of propylene oxide amounted to 14 million kg, and exports are estimated to have been 23 million kg.

Propylene oxide is also produced in Canada, Japan and several European countries, including Belgium, Federal Republic of Germany, France, Italy, The Netherlands, Poland, Spain and UK. In 1973, European propylene oxide capacity was estimated to be 903 million kg. This compound has been produced commercially in Japan since 1960; in 1974, the seven producing companies had a total output of 131 million kg.

The widest use for propylene oxide (accounting for 64% of US consumption in 1972) is as an intermediate in the production of polyether polyols, which are used primarily to make polyurethane foams. Much of the remainder

(25%) is used to produce propylene glycol, most of which is consumed in the manufacture of unsaturated polyester resins. Miscellaneous uses, including conversion to dipropylene glycol, glycol ethers and synthetic glycerin, account for the remainder.

Propylene oxide has been used as a fumigant for sterilizing materials ranging from plastic medical instruments to foodstuffs. In the US, propylene oxide is registered for treatment of packaged dried prunes and glacé fruits such as candied cherries; a residue tolerance of 700 mg/kg (expressed as propylene glycol) has been set down. It is also registered as an insecticidal and fungicidal fumigant for cocoa, gums, processed spices, starch and processed nut meats (except peanuts) when such bulk foods are to be further processed into a final food. The residue tolerance for products so treated is 300 mg/kg (expressed as propylene oxide) (US Code of Federal Regulations, 1975). This compound may also be used for sterilizing foodstuffs such as spices, cocoa, flour, dried egg powder, desiccated coconut, dried fruits and dehydrated vegetables (Wesley et al., 1965).

Permissible levels of propylene oxide in the working environment have been established in various countries (Winell, 1975). The threshold limit value in the US is 240 mg/m^3 (100 ppm); the maximum allowable concentration in the USSR is 1 mg/m^3.

2.2 Occurrence

Several studies have been made on the persistence of propylene oxide in treated foods. When various foods (including cereal flours, sugars, dried fish, milk powder, seasonings, dried fruits, biscuits, etc.) were fumigated with 2:8 propylene oxide:carbon dioxide for 2-4 hours at 50°C, a propylene oxide residue was detected by gas chromatography in all samples except sucrose, glucose, table salt and sodium glutamate. Levels of 1000-2600 mg/kg were found in nutmeg, pepper and coriander; dried fish, wheat and soya bean flours contained the lowest amounts of residue (Oguma et al., 1968). Levels of 4000-9000 mg/kg propylene oxide were found in samples of linseed, soya bean, sesame, rapeseed, olive and castor oils, in lard, beef tallow, butter, mayonnaise and shortening, and in linoleic and oleic acids after fumigation at 50°C for 2 hours. When the fumigated fatty materials were kept at 37°C for 24 hours, no propylene oxide was found in linseed, soya bean and olive oils, but 4147 mg/kg were found in lard and 5910 mg/kg in oleic acid (Oguma *et al.*, 1969).

Various plastic and cellulose products used as food wrappings and containers were fumigated with a 2:8 combination of propylene oxide and carbon dioxide. The fumigant residue detected by gas chromatography immediately, or after storage for 3 hours at room temperature, was more than 2000 mg/kg in cellulose acetate film, wood shavings, paper cups, rubber tubing, nylon film, polycarbonate film and polyvinylidene chloride film. Some polyethylene products contained more than 1500 mg/kg propylene oxide (Hirashima *et al.*, 1970).

2.3 Analysis

Propylene oxide can be determined volumetrically (Gunther, 1965; Swan, 1954) and by gas chromatography in various foods (Heuser & Scudamore, 1969; Oguma *et al.*, 1968, 1969), in plastic and cellulose products (Hirashima *et al.*, 1970) and in a mixture of lower olefin oxides and aldehydes (Kaliberdo & Vaabel, 1967). It can be measured in air samples by spectrophotometry (Pozzoli *et al.*, 1968; Salyamon, 1969); nanomole quantities can be determined by measurement of residual periodate after formation of glycol and subsequent cleavage with periodate (Mishmash & Meloan, 1972).

3. Biological Data Relevant to the Evaluation of Carcinogenic Risk to Man

3.1 Carcinogenicity and related studies in animals

Subcutaneous and/or intramuscular administration

Rat: Of 12 rats (age at start not specified) given total doses of 1500 mg/kg bw propylene oxide in arachis oil by s.c. injection within 325 days (dosing schedule not specified), 8 developed local sarcomas after 507-739 days. In a similar experiment in which total doses of 1500 mg/kg bw propylene oxide in water were injected subcutaneously, 1/12 rats developed a local sarcoma after 158 days, and 2 developed local sarcomas after 737 days. In a concurrent experiment, ethylene oxide produced negative results (Walpole, 1958).

3.2 Other relevant biological data

(a) Experimental systems

The LD_{50}'s of propylene oxide given intragastrically to rats and guinea-pigs were 1.14 and 0.69 g/kg bw, respectively (Smyth et al., 1941); the percutaneous LD_{50} in rabbits was 1.3 g/kg bw (Weil et al., 1963).

Rats tolerated exposure by inhalation to 9520 mg/m^3 (4000 ppm) of vapour for 0.5 hour, to 4760 mg/m^3 (2000 ppm) for 2 hours, or to 2390 mg/m^3 (1000 ppm) for 7 hours; 4/10 rats died after exposure to the highest concentration after 4 hours. Repeated oral doses of 0.2 g/kg bw administered as a 10% solution in oil on 5 days/week for 24 days produced no toxic effects in rats. When guinea-pigs, monkeys, rabbits and rats were exposed for 7 hours to propylene oxide vapour on 5 days/week for 6 or 7 months, rabbits and monkeys, but not guinea-pigs or rats, tolerated 1095 mg/m^3 (460 ppm). While monkeys, rabbits, rats and male guinea-pigs tolerated 464 mg/m^3 (195 ppm) propylene oxide vapour, in female guinea-pigs there was an increase in the average weight of lungs; all four species tolerated 243 mg/m^3 (102 ppm) without adverse effects (Rowe et al., 1956). Propylene oxide is about one-third as toxic as ethylene oxide when administered by ingestion or by inhalation, in all of the species studied.

In rabbits, hyperaemia and oedema of the shaved skin resulted from contact with undiluted or aqueous solutions of propylene oxide. Exposure of rats and guinea-pigs to propylene oxide vapour produced eye irritation, nasal irritation, difficulty in breathing, drowsiness and weakness (Rowe et al., 1956).

Propylene oxide reacts with DNA at neutral pH to yield two principal products, N-7-(2-hydroxypropyl)guanine and N-3-(2-hydroxypropyl)adenine (Lawley & Jarman, 1972).

Reverse mutations were induced in macroconidia of the purple, adenine-requiring mutant 38701 of *Neurospora crassa* after treatment with 0.5 M propylene oxide in water for 15 minutes (Kølmark & Giles, 1955). Propylene oxide has also induced recessive lethal mutations in *Drosophila melanogaster* (Rapoport, 1948a,b; Schalet, 1954).

(b) Man

Three cases of corneal burns from propylene oxide vapour were described by McLaughlin (1946).

3.3 Observations in man

No data were available to the Working Group.

4. Comments on Data Reported and Evaluation[1]

4.1 Animal data

Propylene oxide was carcinogenic in a limited study in rats by subcutaneous injection: it produced local sarcomas.

4.2 Human data

No case reports or epidemiological studies were available to the Working Group.

---

[1] See also the section 'Animal Data in Relation to the Evaluation of Risk to Man' in the introduction to this volume, p. 17.

5. References

Gunther, D.A. (1965) Determination of adsorbed ethylene and propylene oxides by distillation and titration. Analyt. Chem., 37, 1172-1173

Heuser, S.G. & Scudamore, K.A. (1969) Determination of fumigant residues in cereals and other foodstuffs: a multi-detection scheme for gas chromatography of solvent extracts. J. Sci. Fd Agric., 20, 566-572

Hirashima, T., Oguma, T., Hosogai, Y. & Fujii, S. (1970) Gaseous antimicrobal agents. III. Determination of propylene oxide residue in food wrappings and containers. J. Fd hyg. Soc. Japan, 11, 161-163

Kaliberdo, L.M. & Vaabel, A.S. (1967) Quantitative determination of lower olefin oxides in their mixture with aldehydes by gas-liquid chromatography. Zh. analyt. Khim., 22, 1590-1592

Kølmark, G. & Giles, N.H. (1955) Comparative studies of monoepoxides as inducers of reverse mutations in *Neurospora*. Genetics, 40, 890-902

Lawley, P.D. & Jarman, M. (1972) Alkylation by propylene oxide of deoxyribonucleic acid, adenine, guanosine and deoxyguanylic acid. Biochem. J., 126, 893-900

Mark, H.F., Gaylord, N.G. & Bikalis, N.M., eds (1967) Encyclopedia of Polymer Science and Technology, Vol. 6, Plastics, Resins, Rubbers, Fibers, New York, Interscience, p. 146

McLaughlin, R.S. (1946) Chemical burns of the human cornea. Amer. J. Ophthal., 29, 1355-1362

Mishmash, H.E. & Meloan, C.E. (1972) Indirect spectrophotometric determination of nanomole quantities of oxiranes. Analyt. Chem., 44, 835-836

Oguma, T., Hosogai, Y., Fujii, S. & Kawashiro, I. (1968) Gaseous antimicrobial agents. I. Determination of propylene oxide residue in foods. J. Fd hyg. Soc. Japan, 9, 395-398

Oguma, T., Hosogai, Y. & Fujii, S. (1969) Gaseous antimicrobial agents. II. Determination of propylene oxide residue in fats and oils. J. Fd hyg. Soc. Japan, 10, 37-39

Pozzoli, L., Bobbio, G. & Armeli, G. (1968) Spectrophotometric determination of ethylene and propylene oxides and ethyl and butyl alcohols in air. Lav. umano, 20, 409-417

Preussmann, R., Schneider, H. & Epple, F. (1969) Untersuchungen zum Nachweis alkylierender Agentien. II. Der Nachweis verschiedener Klassen alkylierender Agentien mit einer Modifikation der Farbreaktion mit 4-(4'-Nitrobenzyl)pyridin (NBP). Arzneimittelforsch., 19, 1059-1073

Ragelis, E.P., Fisher, B.S. & Klimeck, B.A. (1966) Note on determination of chlorohydrins in foods fumigated with ethylene oxide and with propylene oxide. J. Ass. off. analyt. Chem., 49, 963-965

Rapoport, I.A. (1948a) Alkylation of gene molecule. Dokl. Akad. Nauk SSR, 59, 1183-1186

Rapoport, I.A. (1948b) Action of ethylene oxide, glycidol and glycols on gene mutation. Dokl. Akad. Nauk SSR, 60, 469-472

Rowe, V.K., Hollingsworth, R.L., Oyen, F., McCollister, D.D. & Spencer, H.C. (1956) Toxicity of propylene oxide determined on experimental animals. Arch. industr. Hlth, 13, 228-236

Salyamon, G.S. (1969) Determination of propylene oxide in the air. Gig. i Sanit., 34, 51-53

Schalet, A. (1954) The mutagenic action of 1,2-propylene oxide and ethyl sulfate on mature sperm. *Drosophila* Information Service 28, Part 2: Notes, Bibliography, Directory, Eugene, Oregon, University of Oregon, p. 15

Smyth, H.F., Jr, Seaton, J. & Fischer, L. (1941) The single dose toxicity of some glycols and derivatives. J. industr. Hyg. Toxicol., 23, 259-268

Stecher, P.G., ed. (1968) The Merck Index, 8th ed., Rahway, NJ, Merck & Co., p. 877

Swan, J.D. (1954) Determination of epoxides with sodium sulfite. Analyt. Chem., 26, 878-880

US Code of Federal Regulations (1975) Propylene oxide. Food and Drugs, Title 21, Part 123.380, Washington DC, US Government Printing Office, p. 677

US International Trade Commission (1975) Synthetic Organic Chemicals, US Production and Sales, 1973, ITC Publication 728, Washington DC, US Government Printing Office, p. 205

US Tariff Commission (1926) Census of Dyes and Other Synthetic Organic Chemicals, 1925, Tariff Information Series No. 26, Washington DC, US Government Printing Office, p. 147

Walpole, A.L. (1958) Carcinogenic action of alkylating agents. Ann. N.Y. Acad. Sci., 68, 750-761

Weil, C.S., Condra, N., Haun, C. & Striegel, J.A. (1963) Experimental carcinogenicity and acute toxicity of representative epoxides. Amer. industr. Hyg. Ass. J., 24, 305-325

Wesley, F., Rourke, B. & Darbishire, O. (1965) The formation of persistent toxic chlorohydrins in foodstuffs by fumigation with ethylene oxide and with propylene oxide. J. Fd Sci., 30, 1037-1042

Winell, M.A. (1975) An international comparison of hygienic standards for chemicals in the work environment. Ambio, 4, 34-36

STYRENE OXIDE*

1. Chemical and Physical Data

1.1 Synonyms and trade names

Chem. Abstr. Reg. Serial No.: 96-09-3

Chem. Abstr. Name: Phenyloxirane

Epoxyethylbenzene; (epoxyethyl)benzene; 1,2-epoxyethylbenzene; epoxystyrene; α,β-epoxystyrene; phenethylene oxide; phenylethylene oxide; 1-phenyl-1,2-epoxyethane; 2-phenyloxirane; phenyl oxirane; styrene epoxide; styreneoxide; styryl oxide

1.2 Chemical formula and molecular weight

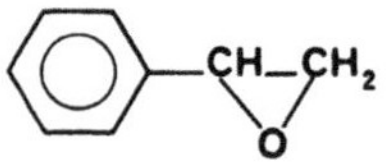

C_8H_8O Mol. wt: 120.2

1.3 Chemical and physical properties

(a) Description: Colourless liquid

(b) Boiling-point: 194.1-195°C

(c) Freezing-point: -36.8°C

(d) Density: d_{20}^{20} 1.0540

(e) Refractive index: n_D^{25} 1.5328

(f) Spectroscopy data: λ_{max} 250 nm; $E_1^1 = 13.2$

(g) Solubility: Miscible with water (0.28 w/w at 25°C); miscible with most organic solvents

---

*Considered by the Working Group, February 1976

(h) <u>Volatility</u>: Vapour pressure is 0.3 mm at 20°C.

(i) <u>Reactivity</u>: Polymerizes and reacts with active hydrogen compounds (e.g., alcohols, amines). Reacts with 4-(4'-nitrobenzyl)pyridine (Preussmann *et al.*, 1969)

1.4 Technical products and impurities

Styrene oxide (98 mole % pure) is available in the US with the following specifications: density, 1.0490-1.0515 (25/25°C); distillation range at 760 mm: fraction between 5 and 95% by volume shall boil within a 3.0°C range, which includes the temperature 194.1°C; water, 0.25% by wt (Mark *et al.*, 1967).

2. Production, Use, Occurrence and Analysis

For important background information on this section, see preamble, p. 19.

2.1 Production and use

Styrene oxide was prepared in 1905 from α-phenyl-β-iodoethanol by treatment with potassium hydroxide (Fourneau & Tiffeneau, 1905). It is reported to be produced commercially either by the chlorohydrin route or by epoxidation of styrene with peroxyacetic acid (Lapkin, 1967).

Styrene oxide is produced in the US by one company at two locations. In Japan, one company has been producing this compound commercially since 1964. Annual production has approached 100 thousand kg in the past, but smaller quantities are now being produced.

Styrene oxide is used as a reactive diluent in epoxy resins (Lee & Neville, 1967). It is also reported to be useful as an intermediate in the preparation of agricultural and biological chemicals, cosmetics, surface coatings and in the treatment of textiles and fibres.

In Japan, styrene oxide is used primarily as an intermediate for the production of phenylethyl alcohol and as a diluent in epoxy resins.

2.2 Occurrence

No data were available to the Working Group.

2.3 Analysis

Styrene oxide can be determined volumetrically in epoxide-glycol mixtures (Swan, 1954). It has been analysed in biological media by gas chromatography with flame-ionization detection and by thin-layer chromatography of the picrate (Leibman & Ortiz, 1970). Indirect spectrophotometric determination of styrene oxide at the nanomole level has also been reported (Mishmash & Meloan, 1972).

3. Biological Data Relevant to the Evaluation of Carcinogenic Risk to Man

3.1 Carcinogenicity and related studies in animals

Skin application

Mouse: Forty 12-week old C_3H mice were painted on the clipped dorsal skin with a 5% solution of styrene oxide in acetone thrice weekly for life. No skin tumours were observed in 33 animals that survived 17-24 months. Forty C_3H mice were similarly painted with a 10% solution of styrene oxide in acetone; only 2 mice survived at 17 months, and no tumours were observed (Weil *et al.*, 1963).

Of 30 8-week old male Swiss ICR/Ha mice given thrice weekly applications of 0.1 ml of a 10% solution of styrene oxide in benzene on the clipped dorsal skin for life, 3 developed skin tumours; one of these had a squamous-cell carcinoma. The median survival time was 431 days. Of 150 benzene-painted controls, 11 developed skin tumours, and one of these had a squamous-cell carcinoma (Van Duuren *et al.*, 1963).

3.2 Other relevant biological data

(a) Experimental systems

The oral LD_{50} of styrene oxide in Wistar rats is 4290 mg/kg bw (Smyth *et al.*, 1954); the i.p. LD_{50} is 460 mg/kg bw (Ohtsuji & Ikeda, 1971); and the 4-hour LC_{50} is 4900 mg/m^3 (1000 ppm) (Weil *et al.*, 1963). The LD_{50} by skin application in male New Zealand rabbits is 1060 mg/kg bw (Smyth *et al.*, 1954).

Styrene oxide causes corneal injury in rabbits even with dilutions as low as 1%. Intradermal injection sensitized 6 of 11 guinea-pigs (Weil *et al.*, 1963).

The main route of excretion of styrene oxide metabolites in animals is urinary; in rabbits, about 80% of a single oral dose was excreted *via* the kidneys (James & White, 1967).

Analysis of urine from rabbits given 1.7 mmol/kg bw styrene oxide (1) (see scheme) revealed 1.2% *N*-acetyl-*S*-(2-hydroxyphenethyl)-L-cysteine (hydroxyphenethyl mercapturic acid) (2), 30% (+)-mandelic acid (4), 25% hippuric acid (5) and 20% glucosiduronic acid; a greater proportion (6%) of *N*-acetyl-*S*-(2-hydroxyphenethyl)-L-cysteine (2) was excreted by rats given 2.1 mmol/kg bw. Phenylethylene glycol (3) *per se* was not identified amongst the urinary metabolites of styrene oxide (1) (James & White, 1967). This evidence is corroborated by the finding of Ohtsuji & Ikeda (1971) that in rats styrene oxide (1) and phenylethylene glycol (3) yielded phenyl-glyoxylic acid (6), mandelic acid (4) and hippuric acid (5). Injection of mandelic acid into rats resulted in the excretion of increased amounts of phenylglyoxylic acid (6), hippuric acid (5) and mandelic acid (4) in the urine; but administration of phenylglyoxylic acid (6) failed to produce any compound other than phenylglyoxylic acid (6) itself. It is improbable that mandelic acid (4) and phenylglyoxylic acid (6) are interconvertible *in vivo* (Ohtsuji & Ikeda, 1971).

The first step in the formation of *N*-acetyl-*S*-(2-hydroxyphenethyl)-L-cysteine (2) is catalysed by glutathione-*S*-epoxide transferase (James & White, 1967). Conjugation of the epoxide with glutathione was demonstrated *in vitro* in rat liver cytosol (Boyland & Williams, 1965) and in a purified enzyme preparation (Fjellstedt *et al.*, 1973). Leibman & Ortiz (1970) demonstrated that styrene oxide is metabolized into phenylethylene glycol (3) by hepatic microsomal preparations in the absence of a NADPH-generating system.

Styrene oxide (1) is converted *in vitro* into styrene glycol (phenyl-ethylene glycol) (3) by microsomal epoxide hydrase from the liver, kidneys, intestine, lungs and skin of several mammalian species (Oesch, 1973).

Scheme

(2) N-Acetyl-S-(2-hydroxyphenethyl)-L-cysteine: Ph–CH(OH)–CH$_2$–S–CH$_2$–CH(NH–CO–CH$_3$)–COOH

(1) Styrene oxide: Ph–CH(–O–)CH$_2$ (epoxide)

(3) Styrene glycol (phenylethyleneglycol): Ph–CH(OH)–CH$_2$OH

(4) Mandelic acid: Ph–CH(OH)–COOH

Benzoic acid: Ph–COOH

(6) Phenylglyoxylic acid: Ph–CO–COOH

(5) Hippuric acid: Ph–CO–NH–CH$_2$–COOH

Metabolic pathways for styrene oxide

The biotransformation of styrene oxide into phenylethylene glycol was stimulated by pre-treatment of rats with phenobarbitone; however, the further metabolism of phenylethylene glycol to mandelic acid was not (Oesch *et al.*, 1971; Ohtsuji & Ikeda, 1971).

Styrene oxide caused 18% inhibition of the growth of Walker carcinoma in rats (Hendry *et al.*, 1951).

It produced reverse mutations in *Salmonella typhimurium* strains TA1535 and TA100 (Milvy & Garro, 1976), forward mutations in *Schizosaccharomyces pombe*, mitotic gene conversions in strain D4 of *Saccharomyces cerevisiae* and azaguanine-resistant mutants in V79 hamster cells (Loprieno *et al.*, 1976).

(b) Man

Acute exposure to styrene oxide causes skin and eye irritation and skin sensitization. There is some evidence that it is absorbed slowly through the skin (Hine & Rowe, 1963).

Urine of workers exposed to styrene oxide vapour contained large amounts of mandelic acid (4) and phenylglyoxylic acid (6) (Huzl *et al.*, 1967; Ohtsuji & Ikeda, 1970), but the hippuric acid (5) concentrations were normal (Ohtsuji & Ikeda, 1970; Stewart *et al.*, 1968).

3.3 Observations in man

No data were available to the Working Group.

4. Comments on Data Reported and Evaluation

4.1 Animal data

Styrene oxide has been tested in two limited studies in mice by skin application. No significant increase in the incidence of skin tumours was observed.

4.2 Human data

No case reports or epidemiological studies were available to the Working Group.

5. References

Boyland, E. & Williams, K. (1965) An enzyme catalysing the conjugation of epoxides with glutathione. Biochem. J., 94, 190-197

Fjellstedt, T.A., Allen, R.H., Duncan, B.K. & Jakoby, W.B. (1973) Enzymatic conjugation of epoxides with glutathione. J. biol. Chem., 248, 3702-3707

Fourneau & Tiffeneau (1905) Sur quelques oxydes d'éthylène aromatiques mono-substitués. C.R. Acad. Sci. (Paris), 140, 1595-1597

Hendry J.A., Homer, R.F., Rose, F.L. & Walpole, A.L. (1951) Cytotoxic agents. II. Bis-epoxides and related compounds. Brit. J. Pharmacol., 6, 235-255

Hine, C.H. & Rowe, V.K. (1963) Styrene oxide. In: Patty, F.D., ed., Industrial Hygiene and Toxicology, 2nd ed., Vol. 2, New York, Interscience, pp. 1649-1651

Hůzl, F., Sýkora, J., Mainerová, J., Jankova, J., Šrutek, J., Junger, V. & Lahn, V. (1967) To the problem of health hazard during the work with styrene. Pracov. Lék., 19, 121-124

James, S.P. & White, D.A. (1967) The metabolism of phenethyl bromide, styrene and styrene oxide in the rabbit and rat. Biochem. J., 104, 914-921

Lapkin, M. (1967) Epoxides. In: Kirk, R.E. & Othmer, D.F., eds, Encyclopedia of Chemical Technology, 2nd ed., Vol. 8, New York, John Wiley and Sons, p. 289

Lee, N. & Neville, K. (1967) Handbook of Epoxy Resins, New York, McGraw-Hill, p. 13-10

Leibman, K.C. & Ortiz, E. (1970) Epoxide intermediates in microsomal oxidation of olefins to glycols. J. Pharmacol. exp. Ther., 173, 242-246

Loprieno, N., Abbondandolo, A., Barale, R., Baroncelli, S., Bonatti, S., Bronzetti, G., Cammellini, A., Corsi, C., Corti, G., Frezza, D., Leporini, C., Mazzaccaro, A., Nieri, R., Rosellini, D. & Rossi, A. (1976) Mutagenicity of industrial compounds: vinyl chloride, styrene and their possible metabolites. Mutation Res. (in press)

Mark, N.F., Gaylord, N.G. & Bikalis, N.M., eds (1967) Encyclopedia of Polymer Science and Technology, Vol. 6, New York, Interscience, p. 170

Milvy, P. & Garro, A.J. (1976) Mutagenic activity of styrene oxide (1,2-epoxyethylbenzene), a presumed styrene metabolite. Mutation Res., 40, 15-18

Mishmash, H.E. & Meloan, C.E. (1972) Indirect spectrophotometric determination of nanomole quantities of oxiranes. Analyt. Chem., 44, 835-836

Oesch, F. (1973) Mammalian epoxide hydrases: inducible enzymes catalysing the inactivation of carcinogenic and cytotoxic metabolites derived from aromatic and olefinic compounds. Xenobiotica, 3, 305-340

Oesch, F., Jerina, D.M. & Daly, J. (1971) A radiometric assay for hepatic epoxide hydrase activity with (7-^{3}H) styrene oxide. Biochem. biophys. acta, 227, 685-691

Ohtsuji, H. & Ikeda, M. (1970) A rapid colorimetric method for the determination of phenylglyoxylic acid and mandelic acids. Its application to the urinalyses of workers exposed to styrene vapour. Brit. J. industr. Med., 27, 150-154

Ohtsuji, H. & Ikeda, M. (1971) The metabolism of styrene in the rat and the stimulatory effect of phenobarbitol. Toxicol. appl. Pharmacol., 18, 321-328

Preussmann, R., Schneider, H. & Epple, F. (1969) Untersuchungen zum Nachweis alkylierender Agentien. II. Der Nachweis verschiedener Klassen alkylierender Agentien mit einer Modifikation der Farbreaktion mit 4-(4'-Nitrobenzyl)pyridin (NBP). Arzneimittelforsch., 19, 1059-1073

Smyth, H.F., Jr, Carpenter, C.P., Weil, C.S. & Pozzani, U.C. (1954) Range-finding toxicity data, list V. Arch. industr. Hyg. occup. Med., 10, 61-68

Stewart, R.D., Dodd, H.C., Baretta, E.D. & Schaffer, A.W. (1968) Human exposure to styrene vapour. Arch. environm. Hlth, 16, 656-662

Swan, J.D. (1954) Determination of epoxides with sodium sulfite. Analyt. Chem., 26, 878-880

Van Duuren, B.L., Nelson, N., Orris, L., Palmes, E.D. & Schmitt, F.L. (1963) Carcinogenicity of epoxides, lactones and peroxy compounds. J. nat. Cancer Inst., 31, 41-55

Weil, C.S., Condra, N., Huhn, C. & Striegel, J.A. (1963) Experimental carcinogenicity and acute toxicity of representative epoxides. Amer. industr. Hyg. Ass. J., 24, 305-325

TRIETHYLENE GLYCOL DIGLYCIDYL ETHER*

1. Chemical and Physical Data

1.1 Synonyms and trade names

Chem. Abstr. Reg. Serial No.: 1954-28-5

Chem. Abstr. Name: 2,2'-(2,5,8,11-tetraoxa-1,12-dodecane diyl)bis-oxirane

1,2-Bis[2-(2,3-epoxypropoxy)ethoxy]ethane; 1,2:15,16-diepoxy-4,7,10,13-tetraoxahexadecane; TDE

Epodyl; Ethoglucid; Etoglucide

1.2 Chemical formula and molecular weight

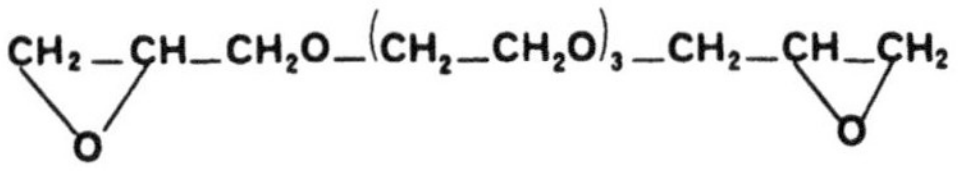

$$CH_2-CH-CH_2O-(CH_2-CH_2O)_3-CH_2-CH-CH_2$$
$$\underset{O}{\diagdown\diagup} \qquad\qquad\qquad\qquad \underset{O}{\diagdown\diagup}$$

$C_{12}H_{22}O_6$ Mol. wt: 262.3

1.3 Chemical and physical properties

(a) Description: Liquid

(b) Boiling-point: 133-149°C at 0.1 mm; 195-197°C at 2 mm

(c) Melting-point: -15 to -11°C

(d) Density: d_4^{20} 1.1312

(e) Refractive index: n_D^{20} 1.4622

(f) Solubility: Miscible with water

(g) Stability: Unstable when exposed to air

---

*Considered by the Working Group, February 1976

1.4 Technical products and impurities

The undiluted compound is available in ampoules of 1 ml (ICI, 1971) or 5 ml (ICI, undated). No data on impurities were available to the Working Group.

2. Production, Use, Occurrence and Analysis

For important background information on this section, see preamble, p. 19.

2.1 Production and use

Triethylene glycol diglycidyl ether was prepared in 1962 by the reaction of epichlorohydrin with triethylene glycol in the presence of a boron trifluoride-diethyl ether complex or by the reaction of triethylene glycol diallyl ether with sodium hypochlorite (Stecher, 1968). It has also been prepared by the reaction of epichlorohydrin with triethylene glycol in the presence of sodium hydroxide (Blyakhman, 1967).

No evidence was found that triethylene glycol diglycidyl ether has ever been produced commercially or found use other than as a research chemical in the US; however, it is manufactured on a commercial scale in the UK for use as an anti-neoplastic agent given by intravenous or intraarterial injection (ICI, 1971; Societé Suisse de Pharmacie, 1975). The drug has also been used in patients with non-invasive carcinoma (multiple papillomatosis of the bladder by direct intracavitary instillation of 100 ml/day of a 1% solution for 2 weeks (Abbassian & Wallace, 1966; ICI, 1971; Riddle & Wallace, 1971). It may be injected into the pleural or peritoneal cavity of patients with malignant effusions, but it is not active orally (ICI, 1971).

Although patents for the use of triethylene glycol diglycidyl ether as a chemical intermediate (e.g., for polymer and fibre modification or in the synthesis of antistatic agents) have been filed, it has probably never been used for this purpose.

2.2 Occurrence

No data were available to the Working Group.

2.3 Analysis

An analytical method for determination of triethylene glycol diglycidyl ether in blood is based on the reaction of the epoxy groups with 4-hydroxy-4'-sulphoazobenzene to give a coloured product with an absorption peak at

440 nm; the limit of detection was 5 µg/ml (Duncan & Snow, 1962). See also section 'General Remarks on the Substances Considered', p. 29.

3. Biological Data Relevant to the Evaluation of Carcinogenic Risk to Man

3.1 Carcinogenicity and related studies in animals

Intraperitoneal administration

Mouse: Five groups of 15 male and 15 female 4-6-week old A/J mice, were given i.p. injections of 0.2 ml of an aqueous solution of triethylene glycol diglycidyl ether thrice weekly for 4 weeks (total doses, 7.2, 3.6, 0.9, 0.22 or 0.06 g/kg bw). When the experiment was terminated, 39 weeks after the first injection, pulmonary tumours were observed in 12/17 (70%, 1.2 tumours per mouse), 9/24 (38%, 0.6 tumours per mouse), 14/29 (48%, 0.6 tumour per mouse), 14/28 (50%, 0.6 tumour per mouse), and 4/29 (14%, 0.1 tumour per mouse) animals, respectively. In 339 male and female controls injected with water only, the pulmonary tumour incidences were 37% in males and 27% in females, and the mean values were 0.5 tumour per mouse in males and 0.3 tumour per mouse in females (Shimkin *et al.*, 1966) [The increased incidence of lung tumours at the highest dose level was highly significant, $P<0.001$].

3.2 Other relevant biological data

(a) Experimental systems

The i.v. LD_{50} of triethylene glycol diglycidyl ether in rats is approximately 700 mg/kg bw; deaths occurred within 2 or 3 days; doses of 1200 mg/kg bw caused death within a few hours. Rats and dogs given i.v. doses of 800 and 500 mg/kg bw, respectively, showed necrosis of the renal tubular epithelium and of the adrenal cortex and intestinal epithelium; intradermal injection in guinea-pigs produced severe necrosis (ICI, undated).

In dogs, an i.v. dose of 100 to 200 mg/kg bw caused the virtual disappearance of neutrophils from the blood after 9 days. Lymphocyte counts fell to 50% of normal; erythrocytes and platelets remained fairly constant, but the brief appearance of polychromatic and nucleated red cells around day 14 showed that erythropoiesis was slightly affected. Dogs with severe granulocytopenia due to triethylene glycol diglycidyl ether may develop a fulminating septicaemia; in the survivors the blood picture returns to normal within 2 or 3 weeks (ICI, undated).

Testicular atrophy and decreased spermatogenic activity were observed in strain A/J mice 39 weeks after the first of 12 i.p. injections (Shimkin et al., 1966).

Repeated i.v. injections of 300 mg/kg bw at 3-5-day intervals to rats with established 6-7-day old Walker carcinomas resulted in complete suppression of tumour growth in 50% of the animals (ICI, undated).

In rats treated intravenously or subcutaneously with triethylene glycol diglycidyl ether, 75% of the dose was excreted in the urine as triethyleneglycol-bis-2,3-dihydroxypropyl ether, together with a trace of the corresponding mono-diol and two sulphur-containing metabolites, which were provisionally identified as a hydroxy-mercapturic acid and an olefinic mercapturate derived from the hydroxy mercapturate by dehydration. A triethylene glycol diglycidyl ether glutathione conjugate and the corresponding cysteinylglycine and cysteine conjugates were excreted into the bile. When triethylene glycol diglycidyl ether was incubated with rat-liver homogenates, only the cysteinylglycine conjugate was found (James & Solheim, 1971).

(b) Man

The severe kidney damage seen in rats and dogs after administration of this compound has not been observed in human patients; however, haematological depression was produced in cancer patients injected with 150-250 mg/kg bw (ICI, 1971).

Side-effects of this drug include leucopenia in 8 patients and temporary dysuria in 12 (ICI, 1971).

3.3 Observations in man

No data were available to the Working Group.

4. Comments on Data Reported and Evaluation[1]

4.1 Animal data

Triethylene glycol diglycidyl ether was carcinogenic in a limited study in mice by intraperitoneal injection: it increased the incidence of pulmonary tumours.

4.2 Human data

No case reports or epidemiological studies were available to the Working Group.

---

[1]See also the section 'Animal Data in Relation to the Evaluation of Risk to Man' in the introduction to this volume, p. 17.

5. References

Abbassian, A. & Wallace, D.M. (1966) Intracavitary chemotherapy of diffuse non-infiltrating papillary carcinoma of the bladder. J. Urol., 96, 461-465

Blyakhman, E.M. (1967) Formation mechanism for glycidyl ethers of glycols. Zh. org. Khim., 3, 1423-1430

Duncan, W.A.M. & Snow, G.A. (1962) Some observations on triethylene glycol diglycidyl ether, a new tumour-inhibitory alkylating agent. Biochem. J., 82, 8P-9P

ICI (undated) Laboratory & Clinical Studies on Epodyl (Triethyleneglycol diglycidyl ether). A new chemotherapeutic agent for the treatment of advanced malignant disease, Wilmslow, Cheshire, Imperial Chemical Industries Ltd, Pharmaceuticals Division, pp. 1-44

ICI (1971) Epodyl in Bladder Cancer, Macclesfield, Cheshire, Imperial Chemical Industries Ltd, Pharmaceuticals Division, pp. 1-20

James, S.P. & Solheim, E. (1971) Metabolism of triethyleneglycol-bis-2,3-epoxypropyl ether (Epodyl) in the rat. Xenobiotica, 1, 43-53

Riddle, P.R. & Wallace, D.M. (1971) Intracavitary chemotherapy for multiple non-invasive bladder tumours. Brit. J. Urol., 43, 181-184

Shimkin, M.B., Weisburger, J.H., Weisburger, E.K., Gubareff, N. & Suntzeff, V. (1966) Bioassay of 29 alkylating chemicals by the pulmonary-tumor response in strain A mice. J. nat. Cancer Inst., 36, 915-935

Société Suisse de Pharmacie (1975) Index Nominum 1975/6, Zurich, p. 584

Stecher, P.G., ed. (1968) The Merck Index, 8th ed., Rahway, NJ, Merck & Co., pp. 1072-1073

MISCELLANEOUS INDUSTRIAL CHEMICALS

BENZYL CHLORIDE*

1. Chemical and Physical Data

1.1 Synonyms and trade names

Chem. Abstr. Reg. Serial No.: 100-44-7

Chem. Abstr. Name: Chloromethylbenzene

Benzylchloride; (chloromethyl)benzene; chlorophenylmethane; α-chlorotoluene; ω-chlorotoluene; tolyl chloride

1.2 Chemical formula and molecular weight

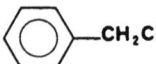

C$_7$H$_7$Cl   Mol. wt: 126.6

1.3 Chemical and physical properties

All from Weast (1975), unless otherwise specified

(a) Description: Colourless liquid

(b) Boiling-point: 179.3°C at 760 mm; 42.6°C at 10 mm

(c) Freezing-point: -39°C

(d) Density: d_{20}^{20} 1.1002

(e) Refractive index: n_D^{20} 1.5391

(f) Spectroscopy data: λ_{max} 217 nm; E_1^1 = 559 (in ethanol)

(g) Solubility: Immiscible with water, but decomposes in hot water; miscible with ethanol, ether and chloroform

(h) Volatility: Vapour pressure is 1 mm at 22°C (Jordan, 1954).

---

*Considered by the Working Group, February 1976

1.4 Technical products and impurities

Benzyl chloride is available in the US as technical and refined grades. Small amounts of sodium bicarbonate or lime are generally added as a stabilizer when it is shipped in steel drums. Other stabilizers which may be used include amines such as triethylamine or dioctylamine, alcohols such as hexyl alcohol and dialkylthioureas (Hawley, 1971; Sidi, 1964).

Typical specifications for commercial benzyl chloride are as follows: clear, colourless liquid; density, 1.104-1.110 at $15.5°/15.5°C$; boiling range of $2°C$ at 760 mm, including $179.4°C$ (Anon., 1970).

2. Production, Use, Occurrence and Analysis

For important background information on this section, see preamble, p. 19.

2.1 Production and use

Benzyl chloride was first prepared by the chlorination of toluene (Canizzaro, 1855); the principal method of commercial production is still the controlled chlorination of toluene until a certain increase in weight is achieved.

Commercial production of benzyl chloride was first reported in the US in 1944 (US Tariff Commission, 1946). In 1972, three US companies reported the production of 36 million kg (US Tariff Commission, 1974); two additional US companies can produce benzyl chloride and may do so for captive consumption. Only minor amounts have been imported or exported by the US.

Benzyl chloride has been produced commercially in Japan since 1936. In 1974, two Japanese companies produced 7.3 million kg, and 83 thousand kg of the chemical were exported. It is produced by one company in Belgium.

It is estimated that 65-70% of the total US production of benzyl chloride is consumed as an intermediate in the manufacture of butyl benzyl phthalate, a vinyl resin plasticizer. The remaining 30-35% is used as an intermediate to produce benzyl alcohol, quaternary ammonium chlorides and a number of other organic chemical products, such as benzyl acetate, benzyl cyanide, benzyl salicylate and benzyl cinnamate.

It has been used as an irritant gas in chemical warfare (von Oettingen, 1955).

Permissible levels of benzyl chloride in the work environment have been established in various countries (Winell, 1975). The threshold limit value in the US is 5 mg/m^3 (1 ppm); the maximum allowable concentration in the USSR is 0.5 mg/m^3.

2.2 Occurrence

No data were available to the Working Group.

2.3 Analysis

Gas chromatography has been used to identify benzyl chloride in a photochlorination study (Solomons & Ratcliffe, 1973) and in trace quantities in water (Junk *et al.*, 1974).

3. Biological Data Relevant to the Evaluation of Carcinogenic Risk to Man

3.1 Carcinogenicity and related studies in animals

(a) Subcutaneous and/or intramuscular administration

Rat: Of 14 14-week old BD rats given weekly s.c. injections of 40 mg/kg bw benzyl chloride in arachis oil for 51 weeks (total dose, 2.1 g/kg bw), 3 developed local sarcomas within 500 days. Of 8 rats given 80 mg/kg bw weekly for 51 weeks (total dose, 3.9 g/kg bw), 6 developed local sarcomas by 500 days; lung metastases were observed in most animals. Injection of arachis oil did not produce local tumours in control rats (Druckrey *et al.*, 1970; Preussmann, 1968).

(b) Intraperitoneal administration

Mouse: Three groups of 20 A/He mice of both sexes, 6-8 weeks old, received 8-12 i.p. injections of benzyl chloride in tricaprylin thrice weekly (total doses, 0.6, 1.5 and 2 g/kg bw). All survivors were killed 24 weeks after the first injection; lung tumours occurred in 4/15, 7/16 and 2/8 surviving mice in the three groups, respectively, with averages of 0.26, 0.50 and 0.25 lung tumours per mouse. The incidence was reported to be not statistically different from that in controls receiving tricaprylin alone or no treatment (Poirier *et al.*, 1975).

3.2 Other relevant biological data

(a) Experimental systems

In rats, the s.c. LD_{50} of benzyl chloride in oil solution is 1000 mg/kg bw (Druckrey et al., 1970). The LC_{50}'s in mice and rats by 2-hour inhalation exposure are 390 and 740 mg/m³ (80 and 150 ppm), respectively (Mikhailova, 1964). Irritation of mucous membranes and conjunctivitis followed exposure to 100-1000 mg/m³ for 2 hours. It is a strong skin sensitizing agent for guinea-pigs (von Oettingen, 1955) and leucopenia has also been observed (Mikhailova, 1964).

Benzyl chloride is absorbed through the lungs and gastrointestinal tract. Following its s.c. injection in rats and rabbits or its oral administration to dogs, it reacts with tissue proteins and is metabolized into benzyl mercapturic acid (N-acetyl-S-benzyl cysteine) (von Oettingen, 1955). Following its oral administration in rabbits it is excreted in the urine as mercapturic acid and benzoic acid (free or conjugated with glycine) (Bray et al., 1958).

Benzyl chloride was weakly mutagenic in strain TA100 of *Salmonella typhimurium* after treatment with 2 mg/plate (McCann et al., 1975).

(b) Man

Air concentrations of 160 mg/m³ (32 ppm) cause severe irritation of the eyes and respiratory tract (von Oettingen, 1955).

3.3 Observations in man

No data were available to the Working Group.

4. Comments on Data Reported and Evaluation[1]

4.1 Animal data

Benzyl chloride was tested in mice by intraperitoneal injection and in rats by subcutaneous injection. It was carcinogenic in rats, in which it produced local sarcomas.

---

[1] See also the section 'Animal Data in Relation to the Evaluation of Risk to Man' in the introduction to this volume, p. 17.

4.2 Human data

No case reports or epidemiological studies were available to the Working Group.

5. References

Anon. (1970) *Monsanto Product Catalog*, 37th ed., St Louis, Missouri, Monsanto Co., pp. 24-25

Bray, H.G., James, S.P. & Thorpe, W.V. (1958) Metabolism of some ω-halogenoalkylbenzenes and related alcohols in the rabbit. *Biochem. J.*, 70, 570-579

Canizzaro, S. (1855) Sur la transformation du toluène en alcool-benzoique et en acide toluique. *Ann. Chim. Phys.*, 45, 468-475

Druckrey, H., Kruse, H., Preussmann, R., Ivankovic, S. & Landschütz, C. (1970) Cancerogene alkylierende Substanzen. III. Alkyl-halogenide, -sulfate, -sulfonate und ringgespannte Heterocyclen. *Z. Krebsforsch.*, 74, 241-270

Hawley, G.G., ed. (1971) *The Condensed Chemical Dictionary*, 8th ed., New York, Van Nostrand-Reinhold, p. 105

Jordan, T.E. (1954) *Vapor Pressure of Organic Compounds*, New York, Interscience, p. 56

Junk, G.A., Richard, J.J., Grieser, M.D., Witiak, D., Witiak, J.L., Arguello, M.D., Vick, R., Svec, H.J., Fritz, J.S. & Calder, G.V. (1974) Use of macroreticular resins in the analysis of water for trace organic contaminants. *J. Chromat.*, 99, 745-762

McCann, J., Spingarn, N.E., Kobori, J. & Ames, B.N. (1975) Detection of carcinogens as mutagens: bacterial tester strains with R factor plasmids. *Proc. nat. Acad. Sci. (Wash.)*, 72, 979-983

Mikhaĭlova, T.V. (1964) Comparative toxicity of chlorous toluene compounds - benzyl chloride, benzal chloride and benzotrichloride. *Gig. Tr. Prof. Zabol.*, 8, 14-19

von Oettingen, W.F. (1955) *The halogenated aliphatic, olefinic, cyclic, aromatic and aliphatic-aromatic hydrocarbons including the halogenated insecticides, their toxicity and potential dangers.* US Department of Health, Education and Welfare, Public Health Service Publication No. 414, Washington DC, US Government Printing Office, pp. 300-302

Poirier, L.A., Stoner, G.D. & Shimkin, M.B. (1975) Bioassay of alkyl halides and nucleotide base analogs by pulmonary tumor response in strain A mice. *Cancer Res.*, 35, 1411-1415

Preussmann, R. (1968) Direct alkylating agents as carcinogens. *Fd Cosmet. Toxicol.*, 6, 576-567

Sidi, H. (1964) Chlorocarbons and chlorohydrocarbons. In: Kirk, R.E. & Othmer, D.F., eds, Encyclopedia of Chemical Technology, 2nd ed., Vol. 5, New York, John Wiley and Sons, pp. 281-289

Solomons, D.A. & Ratcliffe, J.S. (1973) The gas-liquid chromatography of the chloroethanes and chlorotoluenes. J. Chromat., 76, 101-113

US Tariff Commission (1946) Synthetic Organic Chemicals, US Production and Sales, 1972, Report No. 155, Second Series, Washington DC, US Government Printing Office, p. 18

US Tariff Commission (1974) Synthetic Organic Chemicals, US Production and Sales, 1972, TC Publication 681, Washington, DC, US Government Printing Office, p. 20

Weast, R.C., ed. (1975) Handbook of Chemistry and Physics, 56th ed., Cleveland, Ohio, Chemical Rubber Co., p. C-516

Winell, M.A. (1975) An international comparison of hygienic standards for chemicals in the work environment. Ambio, 4, 34-36

β-BUTYROLACTONE*

1. Chemical and Physical Data

1.1 Synonyms and trade names

Chem. Abstr. Reg. Serial No.: 3068-88-0

Chem. Abstr. Name: 4-Methyl-2-oxetanone

3-Hydroxybutanoic acid, β-lactone; 3-hydroxybutyric acid lactone; 3-hydroxybutyric acid, β-lactone

1.2 Chemical formula and molecular weight

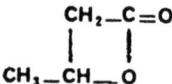

$C_4H_6O_2$ Mol. wt: 86.1

1.3 Chemical and physical properties

(a) Description: Liquid with acetone-like odour (Richter, 1934)

(b) Boiling-point: 54-56°C at 10 mm (Coffey, 1965); 71-73°C at 29 mm; 110-118°C at 180 mm

(c) Density: d_{20}^{20} 1.0555 (Richter, 1934)

(d) Refractive index: n_D^{24} 1.4052 (Van Duuren et al., 1965)

(e) Spectroscopy data: Infra-red band at 1841 cm^{-1} (Coffey, 1965)

(f) Solubility: Miscible with water (15.3% w/w at 18°C) and with most organic solvents (Richter, 1934)

---

*Considered by the Working Group, February 1976

(g) <u>Stability</u>: Stable in acetone and benzene solution for at least 18 days (Van Duuren *et al.*, 1967a)

(h) <u>Reactivity</u>: Hydrolysed by water and aqueous alkali to yield β-hydroxybutyric acid and the salts, respectively

1.4 Technical products and impurities

No data were available to the Working Group.

2. Production, Use, Occurrence and Analysis

For important background information on this section, see preamble, p.19.

2.1 Production and use

β-Butyrolactone can be prepared by the catalytic hydrogenation of diketene (Hasek, 1967). It was produced in Japan from ketene and acetaldehyde until 1973; about 30 thousand kg were produced in that year. It has been used for the production of β-oxybutyryl-*para*-phenetidine.

2.2 Occurrence

No data were available to the Working Group.

2.3 Analysis

No data were available to the Working Group.

3. Biological Data Relevant to the Evaluation of Carcinogenic Risk to Man

3.1 Carcinogenicity and related studies in animals

(a) <u>Oral administration</u>

<u>Rat</u>: Of 5 6-week old female Sprague-Dawley rats given 100 mg/animal β-butyrolactone in 0.5 ml tricaprylin once weekly by gastric intubation, 3 developed squamous-cell carcinomas of the forestomach. The median survival time was 426 days, and the duration of the experiment was 492 days. No forestomach tumours developed in 5 control rats given tricaprylin alone within 587 days; the median survival time was 525 days (Van Duuren *et al.*, 1966).

(b) Skin application

Mouse: Of 30 8-week old female ICR/Ha Swiss mice given 0.1 ml of a 10% solution of β-butyrolactone in benzene thrice weekly on the clipped dorsal skin for life, 21 developed skin carcinomas, the first of which appeared after 346 days, and 4 developed skin papillomas; the median survival time was 466 days. No tumours developed in 60 control animals painted with benzene; the median survival time was 498 days (Van Duuren et al., 1965).

In a similar experiment, 30 female ICR/Ha Swiss mice were treated in the same way with β-butyrolactone in benzene; 20 developed skin papillomas, and of these, 16 developed skin carcinomas. The mean survival time was 438 days. Of 40 female mice of the same strain treated in the same way with a 10% solution of β-butyrolactone in acetone, only 1 developed a skin papilloma at 439 days, which progressed to a carcinoma by 504 days. The median survival time was 452 days, and the duration of the experiment was 598 days (Van Duuren et al., 1967a).

(c) Subcutaneous and/or intramuscular administration

Mouse: Of 50 8-week old female ICR/Ha Swiss mice given weekly s.c. injections of 0.1 mg β-butyrolactone in 0.05 ml tricaprylin for life, 4 developed local sarcomas. The median survival time was 483 days, and the duration of the experiment was 595 days. A second group of 30 mice received 10 mg β-butyrolactone in 0.05 ml tricaprylin weekly; 15 animals developed local fibrosarcomas, and 2 others had local squamous-cell carcinomas. The median survival time was 265 days, and the duration of the experiment was 490 days. No tumours developed in 110 control mice treated with 0.05 ml tricaprylin weekly within 532-581 days (Van Duuren et al., 1966).

Of 16 8-week old female CFW (Swiss Webster) mice given s.c. injections of 0.2 mg β-butyrolactone in 0.1 ml tricaprylin thrice weekly for 4 weeks, 15 were alive at 12 months, and 1 animal developed a local sarcoma. In 16 controls treated with tricaprylin, no local tumours were observed at 18 months (Swern et al., 1970).

Rat: No tumours were seen among 50 6-week old female Sprague-Dawley rats given weekly s.c. injections of 1 mg β-butyrolactone in 0.1 ml tricaprylin;

the median survival time was 559 days. In a further experiment, 20 female rats were given weekly s.c. injections of 100 mg β-butyrolactone in 0.1 ml tricaprylin; 9 animals developed local sarcomas. The median survival time was 283 days, and the duration of the experiment was 533 days. No local tumours were observed in 20 control rats treated with tricaprylin (Van Duuren et al., 1967b).

3.2 Other relevant biological data

No data on the metabolism of β-butyrolactone were available to the Working Group. It inactivates transforming DNA from Bacillus subtilis (Melzer, 1967).

3.3 Observations in man

No data were available to the Working Group.

4. Comments on Data Reported and Evaluation[1]

4.1 Animal data

β-Butyrolactone is carcinogenic in mice by skin application and by subcutaneous injection and in rats by oral administration and by subcutaneous injection. It produced tumours at the site of administration in both species.

4.2 Human data

No case reports or epidemiological studies were available to the Working Group.

---

[1]See also the section 'Animal Data in Relation to the Evaluation of Risk to Man' in the introduction to this volume, p. 17.

5. References

Coffey, S., ed. (1965) Rodd's Chemistry of Carbon Compounds, 2nd ed., Amsterdam, Elsevier, pp. 106-7, 109

Hasek, P.H. (1967) Ketenes. In: Kirk, R.E. & Othmer, D.F., eds, Encyclopedia of Chemical Technology, 2nd ed., Vol. 12, New York, John Wiley and Sons, p. 95

Melzer, M.S. (1967) Effect of carcinogens and other compounds on deoxyribonuclease. Biochim. biophys. acta, 138, 613-616

Richter, R., ed. (1934) Beilsteins Handbuch der Organischen Chemie, 1st Suppl., Vol. 17, Berlin, Springer-Verlag, p. 130

Swern, D., Wieder, R., McDonough, M., Meranze, D.R. & Shimkin, M.B. (1970) Investigation of fatty acids and derivatives for carcinogenic activity. Cancer Res., 30, 1037-1046

Van Duuren, B.L., Orris, L. & Nelson, N. (1965) Carcinogenicity of epoxides, lactones and peroxy compounds. II. J. nat. Cancer Inst., 35, 707-717

Van Duuren, B.L., Langseth, L., Orris, L., Teebor, G., Nelson, N. & Kuschner, M. (1966) Carcinogenicity of epoxides, lactones and peroxy compounds. IV. Tumour response in epithelial and connective tissue in mice and rats. J. nat. Cancer Inst., 37, 825-838

Van Duuren, B.L., Langseth, L., Goldschmidt, B.M. & Orris, L. (1967a) Carcinogenicity of epoxides, lactones and peroxy compounds. VI. Structure and carcinogenic activity. J. nat. Cancer Inst., 39, 1217-1228

Van Duuren, B.L., Langseth, L., Orris, L., Baden, M. & Kuschner, M. (1967b) Carcinogenicity of epoxides, lactones and peroxy compounds. V. Subcutaneous injection in rats. J. nat. Cancer Inst., 39, 1213-1216

γ-BUTYROLACTONE*

1. Chemical and Physical Data

1.1 Synonyms and trade names

Chem. Abstr. Reg. Serial No.: 96-48-0

Chem. Abstr. Name: Dihydro-2(3H)-furanone

γ-BL; 1,4-butanolide; butyric acid lactone; 4-butyrolactone; α-butyrolactone; butyrylactone; butyryl lactone; 4-hydroxybutanoic acid lactone; 4-hydroxybutanoic acid, γ-lactone; γ-hydroxybutyric acid cyclic ester; 4-hydroxybutyric acid lactone; 4-hydroxybutyric acid, γ-lactone; γ-hydroxybutyric acid lactone 6480; BLO(R)

1.2 Chemical formula and molecular weight

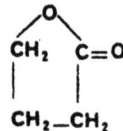

$C_4H_6O_2$ Mol. wt: 86.1

1.3 Chemical and physical properties

From Weast (1975), unless otherwise specified

(a) Description: Oily liquid

(b) Boiling-point: 206°C at 760 mm; 89°C at 12 mm

(c) Melting-point: -42°C

(d) Density: d_0^{16} 1.1286

(e) Refractive index: n_D^{20} 1.4341

---

*Considered by the Working Group, February 1976

(f) <u>Spectroscopy data</u>: λ_{max} 209 nm; E_1^1 = 5 (in methanol); infra-red, ultra-violet, mass and nuclear magnetic resonance spectral data are given by Grasselli (1973).

(g) <u>Solubility</u>: Miscible with water, ethanol, ether, acetone and benzene

(h) <u>Stability</u>: Stable at pH 7; rapidly hydrolysed by bases, slowly hydrolysed by acids

(i) <u>Reactivity</u>: Reacts with inorganic acids and bases, alcohols and amines (Freifeld & Hort, 1967)

1.4 <u>Technical products and impurities</u>

Specifications for a US grade of this compound are as follows: purity, 99.0%; hydroxybutyric acid, 0.1% max.; water, 0.3% max. The purity of another commercial product was reported to be 98.8%, with γ-hydroxybutyric acid, 1,4-butanediol, 1-butanol and water as impurities (Freifeld & Hort, 1967).

2. Production, Use, Occurrence and Analysis

For important background information on this section, see preamble, p. 19

2.1 <u>Production and use</u>

Although γ-butyrolactone can be prepared by a variety of methods (Stecher, 1968), that used for its commercial production in the US is believed to be the dehydrogenation of 1,4-butanediol over a copper catalyst at 200-250°C (Freifeld & Hort, 1967). In Japan, it is produced by the hydrogenation of maleic anhydride (Minoda & Miyajima, 1970). A plant using this process was reported in 1972 to be ready to start production in the UK (Anon., 1972), but no indication was found that this materialized.

Commercial production of γ-butyrolactone was first reported in the US in 1953 (US Tariff Commission, 1954), and one company is still producing at the present time. In 1974, the US imported 33 thousand kg from the UK, 400 kg from Belgium and 300 kg from the Federal Republic of Germany (US Department of Commerce, 1974).

γ-Butyrolactone is produced commercially in the Federal Republic of Germany. Since 1971, approximately 1.5 million kg/year have been made by two Japanese companies, one of which may have stopped production recently. About 180 thousand kg are exported annually, and most of the remaining production is used to manufacture N-methyl-2-pyrrolidone.

US consumption of γ-butyrolactone in 1974 is estimated to have been approximately 14 million kg. It is used principally as a chemical intermediate in the production of 2-pyrrolidone, as an intermediate for other organic chemicals and as a solvent. US consumption of 2-pyrrolidone in that year is estimated to have been about 7 million kg, used primarily as intermediates for vinylpyrrolidone in the manufacture of homo- and copolymers. These polymers are used as film formers in hair sprays, as blood plasma extenders and as clarifying agents in beer and wine; less than 50 thousand kg 2-pyrrolidone were used in 1974 in the production of nylon 4 fibres.

The most important of the other γ-butyrolactone derivatives is N-methyl-2-pyrrolidone; US consumption in 1974 is estimated to have been approximately 5 million kg, used primarily as a solvent (e.g., in the extraction of butadiene and as a polymer solvent). γ-Butyrolactone is also used as an intermediate for the herbicide 4-(2,4-dichlorophenoxy)butyric acid (Anon., 1974).

γ-Butyrolactone is used as a solvent for many polymers (including polyacrylonitrile, polyvinyl chloride, polyvinylcarbazole, polystyrene, polyamides and cellulose acetate), for example, in the textile industry as a spinning and coagulating solvent for polyacrylonitrile. It is a good medium for many chemical reactions and is used as a selective solvent (e.g., for acetylene) in the petroleum industry.

The sodium salt has been used as an anaesthetic (Walkenstein *et al.*, 1964).

2.2 Occurrence

Levels of 2 mg/l γ-butyrolactone have been reported in beer (Spence *et al.*, 1973) and 5-31 mg/l in apple brandy (Rudali *et al.*, 1976). It has been found in other comestibles, such as whey (Ferretti & Flanagan, 1971), vinegar (Kahn *et al.*, 1972), wine (Webb *et al.*, 1964), cooked meats (Liebich *et al.*, 1972; Gordon, 1972), roasted filberts (Sheldon *et al.*, 1972), coffee (Gianturco *et al.*, 1966) and tomatoes (Johnson *et al.*, 1971).

It has been detected in a commercial natural liquid wood smoke preparation (Fiddler *et al.*, 1970) and in tobacco smoke condensate (Neurath *et al.*, 1971).

2.3 Analysis

The determination of γ-butyrolactone in the products mentioned above was carried out by gas chromatography, in most instances coupled with mass spectrometry. A colorimetric method (Guidotti & Ballotti, 1968) and gas chromatography (Giarman & Roth, 1964) have been used for its determination in biological tissues. Thin-layer chromatography has also been used (Schepartz *et al.*, 1972).

3. Biological Data Relevant to the Evaluation of Carcinogenic Risk to Man

3.1 Carcinogenicity and related studies in animals

(a) Oral administration

Mouse: A group of 60 4-week old C3H mice of both sexes received a diet containing 1000 mg γ-butyrolactone per kg of diet for life; a further group of 36 XVII/G mice of both sexes was given 2 mg doses in 0.1 ml water twice weekly for life. In C3H mice, no increases in the incidences of mammary tumours in females or of hepatomas in males were observed compared with those in 54 male and 61 female untreated controls. In treated XVII/G mice, the incidence of lung tumours was 55% (average survival, 571 days) compared with 61% in 44 untreated controls (average survival, 595 days) (Rudali *et al.*, 1976).

Rat: Of 7 weanling male albino rats given 4-6 doses of 100-400 mg/kg bw (total doses, 450-1700 mg/kg bw) γ-butyrolactone by stomach tube for over 7 months and surviving 18-28 months after the first dose, 5 developed tumours, including two pituitary tumours, 2 squamous-cell carcinomas of the jaw and 1 interstitial-cell tumour of the testis. Tumours of the jaw and testis were reported to occur only rarely in control rats of the colony used (Schoental, 1968) [The Working Group noted the small number of animals used and that the product was obtained by distillation of a mixture of γ-butyro-lactone and 4,4'-diaminodiphenylmethane].

(b) Skin application

Mouse: Of 30 8-week old male Swiss ICR/Ha mice painted on the clipped dorsal skin with 0.1 ml of a 10% solution of γ-butyrolactone in benzene thrice weekly for life, 2 developed skin tumours; one of these had a skin carcinoma. The median survival time was 292 days. Among 150 benzene-treated controls, 11 mice developed skin tumours; one of these had a skin carcinoma. Mean survival times in the 4 control groups ranged from 262-412 days (Van Duuren et al., 1963). No increase in tumour incidence was observed in a group of 30 female Swiss ICR/Ha mice painted with 0.1 ml of a 10% solution in acetone thrice weekly for life; the mean survival time was 495 days (Van Duuren et al., 1965).

Among 30 4-week old XVII/G mice of both sexes given repeated skin applications of a 1% solution in acetone twice weekly for life the incidence of lung tumours was 21/30 (70%) (average survival, 601 days) compared with 9/17 (53%) (average survival, 499 days) in acetone-treated controls. No skin tumours were observed (Rudali et al., 1976).

(c) Subcutaneous and/or intramuscular administration

Mouse: No local tumours were observed in a group of 16 female Swiss-Webster mice given 12 s.c. injections of 0.005 mg γ-butyrolactone in 0.1 ml tricaprylin thrice weekly for 4 weeks; 11 mice survived 18 months (Swern et al., 1970) [The small dose used should be noted].

Rat: Five 8-week old male Wistar rats received s.c. injections of 2 mg γ-butyrolactone in oil for 61 weeks and were observed up to 100 weeks. All rats survived, and no tumours were observed (Dickens & Jones, 1961) [In the same experiment, a smaller total dose of β-propiolactone produced a 100% incidence of local tumours].

(d) Other experimental systems

Newborn animals: Of 34 newborn XVII/G mice given s.c. injections of 1 μg γ-butyrolactone on the 1st, 4th and 8th days of life, 18 (53%) developed lung tumours (average survival, 590 days) compared with 27/44 (61%) untreated controls (average survival, 595 days) (Rudali et al., 1976).

3.2 *Other relevant biological data*

The oral LD_{50}'s (14 days) of γ-butyrolactone are 800-1600 mg/kg bw in rats and mice (Fassett, 1963) and 500-700 mg/kg bw in guinea-pigs (Freifeld & Hort, 1967); the i.p. LD_{50} in rats and mice is 200-400 mg/kg bw. The LD_{50} following skin application in guinea-pigs is about 5.6 g/kg bw; no skin sensitization occurred (Fassett, 1963).

γ-Butyrolactone has anaesthetic properties: after i.v. administration to rats it is converted rapidly into γ-hydroxybutyric acid which causes depression of the central nervous system. It is also rapidly hydrolysed to γ-hydroxybutyric acid in blood and liver (Roth & Giarman, 1965). In rats, [1-^{14}C] or [4-^{14}C]-hydroxybutyrate given by inhalation is excreted as $^{14}CO_2$; about 66% of the activity was excreted in 6 hours and an additional 10-20% within 18 hours (Walkenstein *et al.*, 1964).

3.3 *Observations in man*

No data were available to the Working Group.

4. Comments on Data Reported and Evaluation

4.1 *Animal data*

γ-Butyrolactone was tested in mice by oral administration, subcutaneous injection and skin application and in rats by oral and subcutaneous administration. No carcinogenic effects were observed.

4.2 *Human data*

No case reports or epidemiological studies were available to the Working Group.

5. References

Anon. (1972) THF import duty lifted in UK, problems at new ICI plant could be behind temporary exemption. Chemical Age International, October, p. 10

Anon. (1974) Herbicide Handbook, 3rd ed., Champaign, Ill., Weed Science Society of America, pp. 126-128

Dickens, F. & Jones, H.E.H. (1961) Carcinogenic activity of a series of reactive lactones and related substances. Brit. J. Cancer, 15, 85-100

Fassett, D.W. (1963) γ-Butyrolactone. In: Patty, F.A., ed., Industrial Hygiene and Toxicology, 2nd ed., Vol. 2, New York, Interscience, pp. 1824-1825

Ferretti, A. & Flanagan, V.P. (1971) Volatile constituents of whey powder subjected to accelerated browning. J. Dairy Sci., 54, 1764-1769

Fiddler, W., Doerr, R.C. & Wasserman, A.E. (1970) Composition of an ether-soluble fraction of a liquid smoke solution. J. agric. Fd Chem., 18, 310-312

Freifeld, M. & Hort, E.V. (1967) 1,4-Butylene glycol and γ-butyrolactone. In: Kirk, R.E. & Othmer, D.F., eds, Encyclopedia of Chemical Technology, 2nd ed., Vol. 10, New York, John Wiley and Sons, pp. 667-676

Gianturco, M.A., Giammarino, A.S. & Friedel, P. (1966) Volatile constituents of coffee. V. Nature (Lond.), 210, 1358

Giarman, N.J. & Roth, R.H. (1964) Differential estimation of γ-butyrolactone and γ-hydroxybutyric acid in rat blood and brain. Science, 145, 583-584

Gordon, A. (1972) Meat and poultry flavour. The Flavour Industry, September, 445-453

Grasselli, J.G., ed. (1973) Atlas of Spectral Data and Physical Constants for Organic Compounds, Cleveland, Ohio, Chemical Rubber Co., p. B-371

Guidotti, A. & Ballotti, P.L. (1968) Concentrazioni di γ-butirrolattone e di acido γ-idrossibutirrico nell'encefalo del ratto dopo somministrazione di γ-butirrolattone e di γ-idrossibutirrato di sodio per via intraperitoneale ed orale. I. Metodo di dosaggio spettrofotometrico e gas-cromatografico. Boll. Soc. Ital. Biol. sper., 44, 112-116

Johnson, A.E., Nursten, H.E. & Williams, A.A. (1971) Vegetable volatiles: a survey of components identified. II. Chem. & Industr., 23 October, 1212-1224

Kahn, J.H., Nickol, G.B. & Conner, H.A. (1972) Identification of volatile components in vinegars by gas chromatography-mass spectrometry. J. agric. Fd Chem., 20, 214-218

Liebich, H.M., Douglas, D.R., Zlatkis, A., Müggler-Chavan, F. & Donzel, A. (1972) Volatile components in roast beef. J. agric. Fd Chem., 20, 96-99

Minoda, S. & Miyajima, M. (1970) Make γ-BL and THF from maleic. Hydrocarbon Processing, November, pp. 176-178

Neurath, G., Dünger, M. & Küstermann, I. (1971) Untersuchung der 'Semi-Volatiles' des Cigarettenrauches. Beitr. Tabakforsch., 6, 12-20

Roth, R.H. & Giarman, N.J. (1965) Preliminary report on the metabolism of γ-butyrolactone and γ-hydroxybutyric acid. Biochem. Pharmacol., 14, 177-178

Rudali, G., Apiou, F., Boyland, E. & Castegnaro, M. (1976) A propos de l'action cancérigène de la γ-butyrolactone chez les souris. C.R. Acad. Sci. (Paris), 282, 799-802

Schepartz, A.I., Fleischman, R.A. & Cisle, J.H. (1972) Thin-layer chromatographic and spectral properties of certain lactones and related compounds. J. Chromat., 69, 411-415

Schoental, R. (1968) Pathological lesions, including tumors in rats after 4,4'-diaminodiphenylmethane and γ-butyrolactone. Israel J. med. Sci., 4, 1146-1158

Sheldon, R.M., Lindsay, R.C. & Libbey, L.M. (1972) Identification of volatile flavor compounds from roasted filberts. J. Fd Sci., 37, 313-316

Spence, L.R., Palamand, S.R. & Hardwick, W.A. (1973) Identification of C_4 and C_5 lactones in beer. Tech. Quart. Master Brew. Ass. Amer., 10, 127-129

Stecher, P.G. (1968) The Merck Index, 8th ed., Rahway, NJ, Merck & Co., p. 184

Swern, D., Wieder, R., McDonough, M., Meranze, D.R. & Shimkin, M.B. (1970) Investigation of fatty acids and derivatives for carcinogenic activity. Cancer Res., 30, 1037-1046

US Department of Commerce (1974) US Imports of Benzenoid Chemicals and Products; Chemical Elements, Inorganic and Organic Compounds, and Mixtures; and Drugs and Related Products (TSUSA Nos. 401.0200 - 440.0000) for Consumption; IM 146, Schedule 4, Parts 1-3, December, Springfield, Virginia, National Technical Information Service

US Tariff Commission (1954) Synthetic Organic Chemicals, US Production and Sales, 1953, Report No. 194, Second Series, Washington DC, US Government Printing Office, p. 136

Van Duuren, B.L., Nelson, N., Orris, L., Palmes, E.D. & Schmitt, F.L. (1963) Carcinogenicity of epoxides, lactones and peroxy compounds. J. nat. Cancer Inst., 31, 41-55

Van Duuren, B.L., Orris, L. & Nelson, N. (1965) Carcinogenicity of epoxides, lactones and peroxy compounds. II. J. nat. Cancer Inst., 35, 707-717

Walkenstein, S.S., Wiser, R., Gudmunsden, C. & Kimmel, H. (1964) Metabolism of γ-hydroxybutyric acid. Biochim. biophys. acta, 86, 640-642

Weast, R.C., ed. (1975) Handbook of Chemistry and Physics, 56th ed., Cleveland, Ohio, Chemical Rubber Co., p. C-219

Webb, A.D., Gayon, P.R. & Boidron, J.N. (1964) Composition d'une essence extraite d'un vin de V. vinifera (variété Cabernet-Sauvignon). Bull. Soc. chim. Fr., 6, 1415-1420

DINITROSOPENTAMETHYLENETETRAMINE*

1. Chemical and Physical Data

1.1 Synonyms and trade names

Chem. Abstr. Reg. Serial No.: 101-25-7

Chem. Abstr. Name: 3,7-Dinitroso-1,3,5,7-tetraazabicyclo(3.3.1)nonane

Dinitrosopentamethenetetramine; dinitrosopentamethylenetetraamine; dinitroso pentamethylenetetramine; di-N-nitrosopentamethylene tetramine; 3,4-di-N-nitrosopentamethylenetetramine; N,N-dinitrosopentamethylene tetramine; N,N'-dinitrosopentamethylenetetramine; N^1,N^3-dinitrosopentamethylenetetramine; DNPT; 1,5-methylene-3,7-dinitroso-1,3,5,7-tetraazacyclooctane; NSC 73799**

Aceto DNPT 40; Aceto DNPT 80; Aceto DNPT 100; ChKhZ 18; Mikrofor N; Micropor; Opex 80; Unicel ND; Unicel NDX; Vulcacel B-40; Vulcacel BN

1.2 Chemical formula and molecular weight

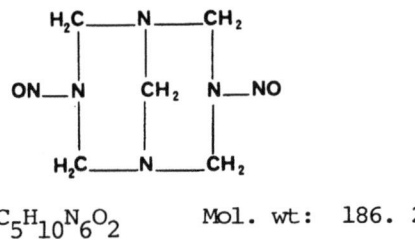

$C_5H_{10}N_6O_2$ Mol. wt: 186.2

1.3 Chemical and physical properties

From Lasman (1965), unless otherwise specified

(a) *Description*: Light-yellow needles

(b) *Melting-point*: 207°C (decomposition)

---

*Considered by the Working Group, February 1976

**Cancer Chemotherapy National Service Centre Number, NCI, NIH, USA

(c) _Solubility_: Slightly soluble in water (about 1%), methanol, ethanol, benzene, ether, acetone and pyridine; readily soluble in dimethylformamide and dimethyl sulphoxide

(e) _Stability_: Violent decomposition occurs in the presence of mineral acids and certain salts (e.g., zinc chloride). Hydrolyses in the presence of dilute hydrochloric acid at 100°C

1.4 Technical products and impurities

Dinitrosopentamethylenetetramine (DNPT) is available in the US as a free-flowing powder in grades containing 99%, 93%, 80% and 42% active ingredient. The inert components of the blended products are inorganic diluents (e.g., silica, clay), processing aids and/or stabilizers (Anon., 1975; Lasman, 1965).

DNPT produced in Japan has the following specifications: purity, greater than 98%; water, less than 0.1%; decomposition temperature, 200-205°C; quantity of gas generated (0°C, 1 atm), 240 ml/g.

2. Production, Use, Occurrence and Analysis

For important background information on this section, see preamble, p. 19.

2.1 Production and use

DNPT can be prepared by the addition of acid to a cold, mixed solution of hexamethylenetetramine and sodium nitrite (Lasman, 1965). Although it was introduced in the US in 1946 by one manufacturer, commercial production was first reported in 1954 (US Tariff Commission, 1955). US consumption of DNPT in 1970 was estimated to have been 1.4 million kg and was projected to be 1.9 million kg in 1975 (Parkinson, 1972).

DNPT is reported to be produced in the Federal Republic of Germany (1 producer), France (3), The Netherlands (1) and the UK (1) (Chemical Information Services Ltd, 1975). Approximately 5 million kg per year are produced in Japan; annual exports are estimated to be approximately 150 thousand kg.

DNPT is used as a nitrogen-releasing chemical blowing agent for the preparation of natural and synthetic unicellular rubber, which is used mainly in carpet underlay, automobile and building weather stripping, thermal insulation material, shoe linings, cushioning and flotation products. DNPT is also an effective blowing agent for the expansion of polyvinyl chloride plastisols and epoxy, polyester and silicone resins.

2.2 Occurrence

No data were available to the Working Group.

2.3 Analysis

Thin-layer chromatography has been used to separate and identify DNPT (Bell & Dunstan, 1966).

3. Biological Data Relevant to the Evaluation of Carcinogenic Risk to Man

3.1 Carcinogenicity and related studies in animals

(a) Oral administration

Rat: In an experiment designed to assess the ability of various chemicals to induce mammary tumours in groups of 20 7-8-week old female Sprague-Dawley rats, a single oral dose of 90 mg/animal DNPT induced no tumours within a six-month period (Griswold et al., 1966) [The short duration of the experiment should be noted].

No tumours were induced in 15 male and 15 female 4-week old Fischer rats given 9 mg/animal by oral gavage on 5 days per week for 1 year and observed for a further 6 months (Weisburger et al., 1966). Hadidian et al. (1968) reported no increases in the incidences of tumours in groups of 12 male and 12 female, 15 male and 15 female and 3 male and 3 female 5-week old Fischer rats, given 0.03, 1, 3 or 9 mg/animal on 4 days/week for 1 year, and observed up to 18 months. A squamous-cell carcinoma of the tongue was seen in a rat given the lowest dose.

(b) Intraperitoneal injection

Rat: A group of 24 6-7-week old male CB rats received weekly i.p. injections of 25 mg DNPT in polyethylene glycol 400 for 26 weeks (total dose, 650 mg) and were observed for up to 2 years. Among 13 rats that survived 16 or more months, 1 developed a hepatoma and 1 a pituitary tumour. One hepatoma was also observed among 24 controls (Boyland et al., 1968).

3.2 Other relevant biological data

In mice, the LD_{50}'s of DNPT are 120 mg/kg bw (i.v.), 130 mg/kg bw (i.p.) and 140 mg/kg bw (s.c.) (Iván, 1965). In rats, the oral LD_{50} is 940 mg/kg bw and the i.p. LD_{50} 220 mg/kg bw. A dose of 80 mg/kg bw given daily by i.p. injection for 30 days was tolerated; higher doses produced toxic effects within the central nervous system, which ranged from depression of conditioned reflexes to tonic and clonic spasms (Desi et al., 1967).

3.3 Observations in man

No data were available to the Working Group.

4. Comments on Data Reported and Evaluation

4.1 Animal data

Dinitrosopentamethylenetetramine was tested in rats by oral administration and intraperitoneal injection. No carcinogenic effects were observed.

4.2 Human data

No case reports or epidemiological studies were available to the Working Group.

5. References

Anon. (1975) Rubber Blue Book, Materials and Compounding Ingredients for Rubber, Rubber World Magazine, New York, Bill Communications, Inc., pp. 314, 316

Bell, J.A. & Dunstan, I. (1966) Thin-layer chromatography of aliphatic nitramines. J. Chromat., 24, 253-257

Boyland, E., Carter, R.L., Gorrod, J.W. & Roe, F.J.C. (1968) Carcinogenic properties of certain rubber additives. Europ. J. Cancer, 4, 233-239

Chemical Information Services, Ltd (1975) Directory of Western European Chemical Producers 1975/1976, Oceanside, NY

Desi, F., Bordás, S., Lehotzky, K. & Hajtman, B. (1967) Investigations on the nervous effects of N,N-dinitroso-pentamethylen-tetramine (Mikrofor) in rats. Med. lavoro, 58, 22-31

Griswold, D.P., Jr, Casey, A.E., Weisburger, E.K., Weisburger, J.H. & Schabel, F.M., Jr (1966) On the carcinogenicity of a single intragastric dose of hydrocarbons, nitrosamines, aromatic amines, dyes, coumarins, and miscellaneous chemicals in female Sprague-Dawley rats. Cancer Res., 26, 619-625

Hadidian, Z., Fredrickson, T.N., Weisburger, E.K., Weisburger, J.H., Glass, R.M. & Mantel, N. (1968) Tests for chemical carcinogens. Report on the activity of derivatives of aromatic amines, nitrosamines, quinolines, nitroalkanes, amides, epoxides, aziridines and purine antimetabolites. J. nat. Cancer Inst., 41, 985-1036

Iván, J. (1965) Pharmacological properties of the analeptic compound N,N'-dinitroso-pentamethylene-tetramine (DNPMT). Acta physiol. hung., 28, 209-216

Lasman, H.R. (1965) Blowing agents. In: Mark, H.F., Gaylord, N.G. & Bikales, N.M., eds, Encyclopedia of Polymer Science and Technology, Vol. 2, New York, Interscience, pp. 555-558

Parkinson, L.G. (1972) The nature of the rubber chemicals market. In: Symposium on Marketing Management and Economics in Rubber Research, Cleveland, Ohio, 1971, American Chemical Society, Division of Chemical Marketing and Economics, New York, Hull & Co., p. 17

US Tariff Commission (1955) Synthetic Organic Chemicals, US Production and Sales, 1954, Report No. 196, Washington DC, US Government Printing Office, p. 125

Weisburger, J.H., Weisburger, E.K., Mantel, N., Hadidian, Z. & Fredrickson, T.N. (1966) New carcinogenic nitrosamines. Naturwissenschaften, 53, 508

1,4-DIOXANE*

1. Chemical and Physical Data

1.1 Synonyms and trade names

Chem. Abstr. Reg. Serial No.: 123-91-1

Chem. Abstr. Name: 1,4-Dioxane

Diethylene dioxide; 1,4-diethylene dioxide; diethylene ether; di(ethylene oxide); 1,4-dioxacyclohexane; dioxan; 1,4-dioxan; *para*-dioxan; dioxane; *para*-dioxane; dioxyethylene ether; glycol ethylene ether; tetrahydro-1,4-dioxin; tetrahydro-*para*-dioxin

1.2 Chemical formula and molecular weight

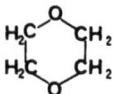

$C_4H_8O_2$ Mol. wt: 88.1

1.3 Chemical and physical properties

(a) Description: Colourless, inflammable liquid

(b) Boiling-point: 101.1°C

(c) Melting-point: 11.8°C

(d) Density: d_4^{20} 1.0329

(e) Refractive index: n_D^{20} 1.4175

(f) Solubility: Miscible with water, organic solvents, aromatic hydrocarbons and oils

(g) Volatility: Vapour pressure is 37 mm at 25°C.

---

*Considered by the Working Group, February 1976

(h) **Stability**: Stable to light but forms explosive peroxide in air, especially in the presence of moisture

(i) **Reactivity**: Reacts with oxygen to form peroxide

1.4 Technical products and impurities

1,4-Dioxane is available in the US in reagent, technical, spectrophotometric and scintillation grades (Hawley, 1971). The technical grade is more than 99.9% pure. Specifications for a typical commercial product are: peroxides (as H_2O_2), 50 mg/kg max.; acidity (as acetic acid), 0.01% by weight max.; water, 0.1% max.; 2-methyl-1,3-dioxolane, 0.05% max.; and non-volatile matter, 0.0025% max. This grade is substantially free from suspended matter (Anon., 1970a).

Specifications for 1,4-dioxane produced in Japan are: purity, 99.99%; boiling-point range, 101-102°C; freezing-point, 11.7°C; density d_4^{20}, 1.0333; and refractive index n_D^{20}, 1.4224. Water is present as an impurity.

2. Production, Use, Occurrence and Analysis

For important background information on this section, see preamble, p. 19.

2.1 Production and use

1,4-Dioxane can be prepared by: (1) the dehydration of ethylene glycol (believed to be the commercial route) (Anon. 1962); (2) the treatment of bis(2-chloroethyl)ether with alkali (Hawley, 1971); or (3) the dimerization of ethylene oxide (Rowe, 1963).

Commercial production of 1,4-dioxane in the US was first reported in 1951 (US Tariff Commission, 1952); production in 1972 was 6.3 million kg (US Tariff Commission, 1974) and in 1973, 7.4 million kg (US International Trade Commission, 1975). There are four companies now producing this compound in the US.

In 1972, three Japanese companies were manufacturing 1,4-dioxane (Anon., 1972a), and another was completing a plant with a capacity of 2.2 million kg per year (Anon., 1972b). In 1968, 600 thousand kg were produced, and in 1973, 2.3 million kg. Japan exported 60-70 thousand kg of 1,4-dioxane in 1974 and about 100 thousand kg in 1975, chiefly to the UK and Australia.

In the US, 1,4-dioxane is used mainly as a stabilizer in chlorinated solvents; in 1973, it was estimated that future growth for this purpose would be 7-8% per year (Anon., 1973). It is also used as a solvent for cellulose acetate, ethyl cellulose, benzyl cellulose, resins, oils, waxes, oil and some dyes (Stecher, 1968), and as a solvent for electrical, agricultural and biochemical intermediates and for adhesives, sealants, cosmetics, pharmaceuticals, rubber chemicals and surface coatings (Anon., 1970b).

The major uses of 1,4-dioxane in Japan are as a solvent, as a surface-treating agent for artificial leather and as a stabilizer for trichloroethylene.

Permissible levels for 1,4-dioxane in the working environment have been established in various countries (Winell, 1975). The threshold limit value in the US is 360 mg/m^3 (100 ppm) and the maximum allowable concentration in the USSR is 10 mg/m^3.

2.2 Occurrence

No data were available to the Working Group.

2.3 Analysis

White *et al.* (1970) used activated-charcoal traps and subsequent gas chromatographic analysis to determine solvent vapours in industrial atmospheres; the same procedure in combination with mass spectrometry was used by Cooper *et al.* (1971). Conditions for separation of a number of solvents, including 1,4-dioxane, by gas chromatography are given by Grupinski (1966). Gas chromatography/mass spectrometry has also been used to determine 1,4-dioxane in water samples (Harris *et al.*, 1974). Reio (1970) used paper chromatography to separate and identify several compounds including 1,4-dioxane. Limits of detection by gas chromatographic methods were of the order of 0.3 µg/l of air.

3. Biological Data Relevant to the Evaluation
of Carcinogenic Risk to Man

3.1 Carcinogenicity and related studies in animals

(a) Oral administration

Mouse: No tumours occurred in groups of 50 male and 50 female B6C3F1 mice administered 0.5 or 1% 1,4-dioxane in the drinking-water for 40-43 weeks (King et al., 1973) [The short duration should be noted].

Rat: A group of 26 male Wistar rats was given 1% 1,4-dioxane in the drinking-water for 63 weeks (total dose, 130 g). Liver tumours, ranging from small neoplastic nodules to multifocal hepatocellular carcinomas, occurred in 6 animals. In addition, 1 rat developed a transitional-cell carcinoma of the kidney pelvis, and 1, a leukaemia. One lymphosarcoma occurred in 9 controls (Argus et al., 1965).

Four groups of 28-32 male Sprague-Dawley rats were given 0.75, 1.0, 1.4 or 1.8% 1,4-dioxane in the drinking-water for 13 months (total doses, 104-256 g/animal) and killed after 16 months. One rat receiving 0.75%, 1 receiving 1.0%, 2 receiving 1.4% and 2 receiving 1.8% 1,4-dioxane developed tumours of the nasal cavity; these were mainly squamous-cell carcinomas, with areas containing adenocarcinomas in 2 cases. Liver-cell tumours (hepatomas and hepatocellular carcinomas) developed in 3 rats receiving 1.4% and in 12 rats received 1.8%. Microscopic lesions described as 'incipient hepatomas' were observed in all treated groups. A subcutaneous fibroma occurred 'on the back of the nose' in 1/30 controls (Argus et al., 1973; Hogh-Ligeti et al., 1970).

Four groups of 60 male and 60 female Sherman rats were given 0, 0.01, 0.1 or 1% 1,4-dioxane in the drinking-water for up to 716 days (daily doses: males, 0, 8-12, 59-113, 914-1229 mg/kg bw; females, 0, 18-20, 130-160, 1416-2149 mg/kg bw). The 50% survival time at the highest dose was 16 months, compared with 22 months in other groups. At the highest level 10 hepatocellular carcinomas, 2 cholangiomas and 3 squamous-cell carcinomas of the nasal cavity were observed, compared with 1 hepatocellular carcinoma in a rat receiving 0.1% 1,4-dioxane. No statistically significant increase in the incidence of tumours was seen in rats given the two lower dose levels (Kociba et al., 1974).

Guinea-pig: Twenty-two male guinea-pigs received drinking-water containing 0.5-2% 1,4-dioxane, such that normal growth was maintained, over 23 months (total dose, 588-623 g/animal). All animals were killed within 28 months. Two animals had carcinomas of the gall bladder, and 3 had hepatomas. No liver tumours were reported in 10 untreated controls (Hogh-Ligeti & Argus, 1970).

(b) Inhalation and/or intratracheal administration

Five groups of 96 male and 96 female Wistar rats were exposed either to air or air containing 0.4 mg/l (111 ppm) 99.9% pure 1,4-dioxane for 7 hours/day on 5 days/week for 2 years. Fifty per cent of the animals survived 20-24 months. No statistically significant increase in the incidence of tumours was observed in the 525 treated rats examined compared with 347 controls (Torkelson et al., 1974).

(c) Skin application

Mouse: Groups of 30 male and 30 female Swiss-Webster mice received thrice weekly paintings of 0.2 ml of an unspecified concentration of 1,4-dioxane in acetone on the clipped dorsal skin for 60 weeks; 1 skin sarcoma and 1 malignant lymphoma were observed. In similar groups of mice, skin paintings were preceded 1 week earlier by application of 50 µg 7,12-dimethylbenzanthracene (DMBA); 4 males and 5 females survived the 59 weeks of treatment. Among 15 mice examined, 8 skin tumours were observed (2 papillomas, 2 squamous-cell carcinomas, and 4 sarcomas); in addition, 24 other tumours (mainly malignant lymphomas and lung tumours) occurred. Eight skin papillomas and 1 malignant lymphoma occurred in 55 animals receiving 50 µg DMBA followed by thrice weekly paintings with acetone alone (King et al., 1973) [The increase in the incidence of skin tumours was significant in the 2-stage skin carcinogenesis experiment ($P<0.01$)].

3.2 Other relevant biological data

(a) Experimental systems

The i.p. LD_{50} of 1,4-dioxane in male Sprague-Dawley rats was 5.6 g/kg bw (Argus et al., 1973). The oral LD_{50}'s in mice, rats and guinea-pigs were 5.7, 5.2 and 3.9 g/kg bw, respectively (Laug et al., 1939). In mice, rats, guinea-pigs and rabbits subjected to repeated 1.5-hour exposures to 3600 mg/m^3 (1000 ppm) 1,4-dioxane in air (total exposures, 78-202.5 hours), vascular congestion of the liver and degenerative changes in the renal cortex were observed (Fairley et al., 1934).

In male rats given single oral doses of 10, 100 or 1000 mg/kg bw ^{14}C-1,4-dioxane, excretion of unchanged 1,4-dioxane in expired air was 0.043 mg/kg bw (0.43%) at the lowest dose and 252 mg/kg bw (25%) at the highest dose (Young & Gehring, 1975).

(b) Man

Exposure of 12 volunteers to a concentration of 1080 mg/m^3 (300 ppm) 1,4-dioxane vapour in air for 15 minutes produced irritation of the eyes, nose and throat (Silverman et al., 1946).

Five acute deaths due to 1,4-dioxane exposure have been reported; haemorrhagic nephritis and liver necrosis were recorded at autopsy (Barber, 1934). Another death, in a worker, probably attributable to one week's exposure to about 1800 mg/m^3 (500 ppm) 1,4-dioxane, has been reported. There was also a possibility of skin absorption, since 1,4-dioxane was used as a solvent to remove glue from hands. Autopsy revealed damage to kidneys, liver and brain (Johnstone, 1959).

3.3 Observations in man

No data were available to the Working Group.

4. Comments on Data Reported and Evaluation[1]

4.1 Animal data

1,4-Dioxane is carcinogenic in rats and guinea-pigs by oral administration: it produced malignant tumours of the nasal cavity and liver in rats and tumours of the liver and gall bladder in guinea-pigs. It was also active as a promoter in a two-stage skin carcinogenesis study in mice. No carcinogenic effect was observed in one inhalation study in rats.

---

[1]See also the section 'Animal Data in Relation to the Evaluation of Risk to Man' in the introduction to this volume, p. 17.

4.2 Human data

No case reports or epidemiological studies were available to the Working Group.

5. References

Anon. (1962) *Dictionary of Commercial Chemicals*, 3rd ed., Princeton, NJ, Van Nostrand, p. 432

Anon. (1970a) *1,4-Dioxane*. Product Information Bulletin No. F-40249B, New York, Union Carbide Corporation

Anon. (1970b) *Product Use Patterns*, New York, Union Carbide Corporation

Anon. (1972a) Dioxane plant in Japan produces 20 tons a month. *Chemical Marketing Reporter*, September 11, p. 18

Anon. (1972b) New dioxane plant completed. *Japan Chemical Week*, April 6, p. 2

Anon. (1973) 1,4-Dioxane. *Chemical Marketing Reporter*, February 5, pp. 11-12

Argus, M.F., Arcos, J.C. & Hoch-Ligeti, C. (1965) Studies on the carcinogenic activity of protein-denaturating agents: hepatocarcinogenicity of dioxane. *J. nat. Cancer Inst.*, 35, 949-958

Argus, M.F., Sohal, R.S., Bryant, G.M., Hoch-Ligeti, C. & Arcos, J.C. (1973) Dose-response and ultrastructural alterations in dioxane carcinogenesis. Influence of methylcholanthrene on acute toxicity. *Europ. J. Cancer*, 9, 237-243

Barber, H. (1934) Haemorrhagic nephritis and necrosis of the liver from dioxan poisoning. *Guy's Hospital Rep.*, 84, 267-280

Cooper, C.V., White, L.D. & Kupel, R.E. (1971) Qualitative detection limits for specific compounds utilizing gas chromatographic fractions, activated charcoal and a mass spectrometer. *J. Amer. industr. Hyg. Ass.*, 36, 383-386

Fairley, A., Linton, E.C. & Ford-Moore, A.H. (1934) The toxicity to animals of 1:4 dioxan. *J. Hyg. (Lond.)*, 34, 486-501

Grupinski, L. (1966) Erfahrungen bei Emissionsmessungen zur Bestimmung von lösemitteldämpfen und Kohlenwasserstaffen. *Wasser, Luft Betrieb*, 10, 77-80

Harris, L.E., Budde, W.L. & Eichelberger, J.W. (1974) Direct analysis of water samples for organic pollutants with gas chromatography-mass spectrometry. *Analyt. Chem.*, 46, 1912-1917

Hawley, G.G., ed. (1971) *Condensed Chemical Dictionary*, 8th ed., New York, Van Nostrand-Reinhold, p. 320

Hogh-Ligeti, C. & Argus, M.F. (1970) Effect of carcinogens on the lung of guinea-pigs. In: Nettesheim, P., Hanna, M.G., Jr & Deatherage, J.W., Jr, eds, Conference on the Morphology of Experimental Respiratory Carcinogenesis, Gatlinburg, Tenn., 1970, AEC Symposium Series No. 21, Springfield, Va., National Technical Information Service, pp. 267-279

Hoch-Ligeti, C., Argus, M.F. & Arcos, J.C. (1970) Induction of carcinomas in the nasal cavity of rats by dioxane. Brit. J. Cancer, 24, 164-167

Johnstone, R.T. (1959) Death due to dioxane? AMA Arch. industr. Hlth, 20, 445-447

King, M.E., Shefner, A.M. & Bates, R.R. (1973) Carcinogenesis bioassay of chlorinated dibenzodioxins and related chemicals. Environm. Hlth Persp., 5, 163-170

Kociba, R.J., McCollister, S.B., Park, C., Torkelson, T.R. & Gehring, P.J. (1974) 1,4-Dioxane. I. Results of a 2-year ingestion study in rats. Toxicol. appl. Pharmacol., 30, 275-286

Laug, E.P., Calvery, H.O., Morris, H.G. & Woodard, G. (1939) The toxicology of some glycols and derivatives. J. industr. Hyg. Toxicol., 21, 173-201

Reio, L. (1970) Third supplement for the paper chromatographic separation and identification of phenol derivatives and related compounds of biochemical interest using a 'reference system'. J. Chromat., 47, 60-85

Rowe, V.K. (1963) Dioxane. In: Patty, F.A., ed., Industrial Hygiene and Toxicology, 2nd ed., Vol. 2, New York, Interscience, pp. 1537-1541

Silverman, L., Schulte, H.F. & First, W.W. (1946) Further studies on sensory response to certain industrial solvent vapors. J. industr. Hyg., 28, 262-266

Stecher, P.G., ed. (1968) The Merck Index, 8th ed., Rahway, NJ, Merck & Co., p. 384

Torkelson, T.R., Leong, B.K.J., Kociba, R.J., Richter, W.A. & Gehring, P.J. (1974) 1,4-Dioxane. II. Results of a 2-year inhalation study in rats. Toxicol. appl. Pharmacol., 30, 287-298

US International Trade Commission (1975) Synthetic Organic Chemicals, US Production and Sales, 1973, ITC Publication 728, Washington DC, US Government Printing Office, p. 199

US Tariff Commission (1952) Synthetic Organic Chemicals, US Production and Sales, 1951, Report No. 175, Washington DC, US Government Printing Office, p. 138

US Tariff Commission (1974) Synthetic Organic Chemicals, US Production and Sales, 1972, TC Publication 681, Washington DC, US Government Printing Office, p. 201

White, L.D., Taylor, D.G., Mauer, P.A. & Kupel, R.E. (1970) A convenient optimized method for the analysis of selected solvent vapors in the industrial atmosphere. J. Amer. industr. Hyg. Ass., 35, 225-232

Winell, M.A. (1975) An international comparison of hygienic standards for chemicals in the work environment. Ambio, 4, 34-36

Young, J.D. & Gehring, P.J. (1975) The dose-dependent fate of 1,4-dioxane in male rats. Toxicol. appl. Pharmacol., 33, 183

ETHYLENE SULPHIDE*

1. Chemical and Physical Data

1.1 Synonyms and trade names

Chem. Abstr. Reg. Serial No.: 420-12-2

Chem. Abstr. Name: Thiirane

2,3-Dihydrothiirene; ethylene episulfide; ethylene sulfide; ethylene episulphide; thiacyclopropane

1.2 Chemical formula and molecular weight

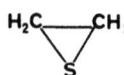

C_2H_4S Mol. wt: 60.1

1.3 Chemical and physical properties

From Weast (1975), unless otherwise specified

(a) Description: Colourless liquid

(b) Boiling-point: 55-56°C (decomposition)

(c) Density: d_4^0 1.0368; d_4^{15} 1.017; d_4^{20} 1.0046

(d) Refractive index: n_D^{20} 1.4937; n_D^{19} 1.490

(e) Spectroscopy data: λ_{max} 258 nm; E_1^1 = 5 (in ethanol); infra-red, ultra-violet and mass spectra are given by Grasselli (1973).

(f) Solubility: Immiscible with water; miscible with ethanol, ether, acetone and chloroform

(g) Volatility: Vapour pressure is 375 mm at 25°C.

(h) Stability: Polymerizes gradually

---

*Considered by the Working Group, February 1976

(i) *Reactivity*: Reacts with 4(4'-nitrobenzyl)pyridine (Preussmann *et al.*, 1969)

1.4 Technical products and impurities

No data were available to the Working Group.

2. Production, Use, Occurrence and Analysis

For important background information on this section, see preamble, p. 19.

2.1 Production and use

Ethylene sulphide was synthesized by the reaction of 2-haloethylthiocyanates with sodium sulphide (Delépine, 1920). Other methods of synthesis include the following: (1) reaction of ethylene carbonate with sodium or potassium thiocyanate; (2) reaction of ethylene monothiocarbonate with sodium carbonate; and (3) reaction of ethylene oxide with thiourea, inorganic thiocyanates or carbonyl sulphide (Gobran, 1969).

Patents have been filed for the use of ethylene sulphide as a monomer (e.g., in the production of homopolymers and copolymers), as a modifying agent for other polymers (e.g., cellulose), as a chemical intermediate (e.g., for pesticides and lubricant additives) and as a direct-acting disinfectant. No evidence was found that it has been used in these applications.

The maximum allowable concentration in the USSR is 0.1 mg/m^3 (Pugaeva *et al.*, 1969).

2.2 Occurrence

Ethylene sulphide has been reported to be a component of a low-temperature distillate of tinned beef (Persson & von Sydow, 1973).

2.3 Analysis

Gas chromatography can be used for the determination of ethylene sulphide (Raulin & Toupance, 1974). Its separation from other sulphides has been discussed by Kremer & Spicer (1973) and Golovnya & Garbuzov (1974).

3. Biological Data Relevant to the Evaluation of Carcinogenic Risk to Man

3.1 Carcinogenicity and related studies in animals

(a) Subcutaneous and/or intramuscular administration

Rat: Two groups of 15 14-week old BD rats received weekly s.c. injections of 8 or 16 mg/kg bw ethylene sulphide in arachis oil for one year, at which time the first tumour appeared in the higher dose group. The animals were observed until death; 4/12 animals given the higher dose developed local sarcomas; 1/15 animals given the lower dose developed a local fibroma. The vehicle was reported to be non-carcinogenic in controls (Druckrey et al., 1970).

3.2 Other relevant biological data

The oral LD_{50} of ethylene sulphide in Wistar rats is 178 mg/kg bw; the i.p. LD_{50} is 42 mg/kg bw; and the LC_{50} during a 30-minute exposure is 10,000 mg/m^3 (4000 ppm) (Brown & Mastromatteo, 1964). The s.c. LD_{50} in BD rats is 90 mg/kg bw (Druckrey et al., 1970). MacFarland et al. (1971) found that the one-hour LC_{50} for ethylene sulphide was 7000 mg/m^3 (2800 ppm), and the 6-hour LC_{50} 1725 mg/m^3 (690 ppm). When given orally, ethylene sulphide is about 6 times as toxic (Brown & Mastromatteo, 1964) as propylene oxide (Smyth et al., 1941).

In rats, the ingestion of high doses of ethylene sulphide caused depression of the central nervous system with unconsciousness (Brown & Mastromatteo, 1964). It is irritating to surface tissues and mucous membranes. Inhalation of this compound caused congestion, oedema and haemorrhage in the lungs (Eisengart, 1967; Kurlyandksy et al., 1966; MacFarland et al., 1971).

Ethylene sulphide induced sex-linked recessive lethals in *Drosophila melanogaster* (Rapoport, 1962).

3.3 Observations in man

No data were available to the Working Group.

4. Comments on Data Reported and Evaluation[1]

4.1 Animal data

Ethylene sulphide was carcinogenic in a limited study in rats by subcutaneous injection: it produced local sarcomas.

4.2 Human data

No case reports or epidemiological data were available to the Working Group.

---

[1]See also the section 'Animal Data in Relation to the Evaluation of Risk to Man' in the introduction to this volume, p. 17.

5. References

Brown, J.R. & Mastromatteo, E. (1964) Acute toxicity of three episulphide compounds in experimental animals. Amer. industr. Hyg. Ass. J., 25, 560-563

Delépine, M. (1920) Sur le sulfure d'éthylène C_2H_4S. C.R. Acad. Sci. (Paris), 171, 36-38

Druckrey, H., Kruse, H., Preussmann, R., Ivankovic, S. & Landschütz, Ch. (1970) Cancerogene alkylierende Substanzen. III. Alkyl-halogenide, -sulfate, -sulfonate und ringgespannte Heterocyclen. Z. Krebsforsch., 74, 241-270

Eisengart, R.S. (1967) Histamine level and histaminopexy of the brain tissues and skin in rats under the effect of industrial poisons. Farmakol. Toksikol., 30, 608-609

Gobran, R.H. (1969) Poly(alkylene sulfides). In: Mark, H.F., ed., Encyclopedia of Polymer Science and Technology, Vol. 10, New York, John Wiley and Sons, pp. 325-336

Golovnya, R.V. & Garbuzov, V.G. (1974) Effect of heteroatom nature on the elution of cyclic sulfur- and oxygen-containing compounds in gas chromatography. Izv. Akad. Nauk SSSR, Ser. Khim., 7, 1606-1608

Grasselli, J.G., ed. (1973) Atlas of Spectral Data and Physical Constants for Organic Compounds, Cleveland, Ohio, Chemical Rubber Co., p. B-931

Kremer, L. & Spicer, L.D. (1973) Gas chromatographic separation of hydrogen sulfide, carbonyl sulfide, and higher sulfur compounds with a single pass system. Analyt. Chem., 45, 1963-1964

Kurlyandksy, B.A., Mashbits, F.D. & Eisengart, R.S. (1966) On the mechanism of non-specific manifestations of chronic poisoning with small amounts of chemical substances. Gig. Tr. Prof. Zabol., 10, 44-49

MacFarland, H.N., Khan, N.R. & Innanen, V.T. (1971) Inhalation toxicity of some aliphatic thiiranes. Bull. environm. Contam. Toxicol., 6, 509-512

Persson, T. & von Sydow, E. (1973) Aroma of canned beef. Gas-chromatographic and mass-spectrometric analysis of the volatiles. J. Fd Sci., 38, 377-385

Preussmann, R., Schneider, H. & Epple, F. (1969) Untersuchungen zum Nachweis alkylierender Agentien. II. Der Nachweis verschiedener Klassen alkylierender Agentien mit einer Modifikation der Farbreaktion mit 4(4'-Nitrobenzyl)pyridin (NBP). Arzneimittelforsch., 19, 1059-1073

Pugaeva, V.P., Klochkova, S.I., Mashbits, F.D. & Eisengart, R.S. (1969) Toxicological assessment and hygienic standard ratings for ethylene sulphide in the atmosphere of industrial premises. Gig. Tr. Prof. Zabol., 13, 47-48

Rapoport, I.A. (1962) Dependence of ethyleneimine mutations on the dose and stage of gametogenesis. Byull. Mosk. Obsh. Isp. Prirody, Otdel Biol., 67, 109-123

Raulin, F. & Toupance, G. (1974) Simultaneous gas chromatographic separation of volatile organic sulphur compounds and C_1-C_4 hydrocarbons. J. Chromat., 90, 218-222

Smyth, H.F., Jr, Seaton, J. & Fischer, L. (1941) The single dose toxicity of some glycols and derivatives. J. industr. Hyg. Toxicol., 23, 259-268

Weast, R.C., ed. (1975) Handbook of Chemistry and Physics, 56th ed., Cleveland, Ohio, Chemical Rubber Co., p. C-508

TRICHLOROETHYLENE*

1. Chemical and Physical Data

1.1 Synonyms and trade names

Chem. Abstr. Reg. Serial No.: 79-01-6

Chem. Abstr. Name: Trichloroethene

Acetylene trichloride; 1-chloro-2,2-dichloroethylene; ethinyl trichloride; ethylene trichloride; trichlorethylene; 1,1,2-trichloroethylene

Algylen; Blancosolv; Chlorylen; Cincosolv; Crawhaspol; Dukeron; Flock Flip; Gemalgene; Germalgene; Threthylen; Threthylene; Trethylene; Trichloran; Trichloren; Triclene; Tri-clene; Trielene; Triklone; Trilene; Triline; Trimar; Triol; Westrosol

1.2 Chemical formula and molecular weight

$$ClCH=CCl_2$$

C_2HCl_3 Mol. wt: 131.4

1.3 Chemical and physical properties

From Weast (1975), unless otherwise specified

(a) Description: Non-flammable, colourless liquid

(b) Boiling-point: 87°C

(c) Melting-point: -73°C; freezing-point: -86.4°C

(d) Density: d_4^{20} 1.4642

(e) Refractive index: n_D^{20} 1.4773

(f) Spectroscopy data: Infra-red, ultra-violet, nuclear magnetic resonance and mass spectra are given by Grasselli (1973).

---

*Considered by the Working Group, February 1976

(g) <u>Solubility</u>: Miscible (0.1% w/v at 20°C) with water (Irish, 1962); miscible with acetone, ethanol, ether and vegetable oils (Lloyd et al., 1975)

(h) <u>Volatility</u>: Vapour pressure is 94 mm at 30°C (Jordan, 1954).

(i) <u>Stability</u>: Slowly decomposed by light with formation of hydrogen chloride

(j) <u>Reactivity</u>: Reacts with sulphydryl groups; subject to autoxidation; not hydrolysed by water under normal conditions

1.4 Technical products and impurities

Trichloroethylene is available in the US in high purity, electronic, USP technical, metal degreasing and extraction grades (Hawley, 1971). Typical analysis of a commercial grade is: boiling range at 760 mm, 86.6-87.8°C; density, d_4^{15} 1.467-1.471; acidity (as HCl), 0.0005% max.; alkalinity (as NaOH), 0.001% max.; no free halogen; residue on evaporation, 0.005% max.; moisture content, not cloudy at -12°C.

Antioxidants, such as amines (0.001 to 0.2%) (Copelin, 1954) or combinations of epoxides and esters (0.2 to 2% total) (Starks, 1956), are added to trichloroethylene.

Specifications for trichloroethylene produced in Japan are: density (20°/20°C), 1.460-1.475; water, not cloudy at 0°C; non-volatile matter, 0.01% max.; acid content (as HCl), 0.003% max.; alkali content (as NaOH), 0.025% max.

2. Production, Use, Occurrence and Analysis

For important background information on this section, see preamble, p. 19.

2.1 Production and use

Trichloroethylene was prepared by Fischer in 1864 during experiments on the reduction of hexachloroethane with hydrogen (Hardie, 1964). The first commercial method for its preparation was the dehydrochlorination of acetylene-derived 1,1,2,2-tetrachloroethane by reaction with calcium hydroxide or by gas-phase pyrolysis. Although this method is still used today, over 90% of the trichloroethylene produced in the US is prepared by the chlorination and dehydrochlorination of ethylene dichloride.

Trichloroethylene has been produced commercially in Austria and the UK since 1908, in Germany since 1910 and in the US since 1925 (Hardie, 1964). Production of trichloroethylene in the US in 1974 was 193 million kg (US International Trade Commission, 1975a); five US companies reported production of 98 million kg during the first nine months of 1975 (US International Trade Commission, 1975b). Output has been decreasing since 1970, when a reported 277 million kg were produced by seven companies (US Tariff Commission, 1972). This decrease in production is due primarily to legislation restricting the use and emissions of trichloroethylene and to the closing of three acetylene-based and one ethylene-based plants.

US exports of trichloroethylene in 1974 were 19 million kg, mostly to Mexico (7.2 million kg), The Netherlands (3.3 million kg), Japan (3.3 million kg) and Brazil (1.4 million kg) (US Department of Commerce, 1975a). Imports during that year totalled 600 thousand kg (US Department of Commerce, 1975b).

In Japan, commercial production of trichloroethylene started in 1935. Four companies produced 90 million kg in 1974, compared to 112 million kg in 1970. In 1973, 2.1 million kg of trichloroethylene were exported.

It was forecast that the world market for trichloroethylene during 1975 would be about 680 million kg (Anon., 1972).

Of the trichloroethylene consumed in the US, about 90% is used for vapour degreasing of fabricated metal parts; another 6% is used as a chain terminator for polyvinyl chloride production; and the remainder is used in a variety of applications. The estimated 1973 Japanese consumption pattern for trichloroethylene was: dry-cleaning, 50%; metal cleaning, 21%; solvent and other uses, 26%; and exports, 3%.

Miscellaneous applications of trichloroethylene include its use as an extractant in food processing (e.g., for decaffeinated coffee), as a solvent in the textile industry and as a chemical intermediate. It has been used as a component in several consumer products, largely because of its solvent properties (Lloyd *et al.*, 1975).

A pharmaceutical grade of trichloroethylene is used as a general anaesthetic in surgical, dental and obstetrical procedures and as an analgesic in the treatment of trigeminal neuralgia. It has been used as a disinfectant and detergent for skin, minor wounds and surgical instruments. It has also been used in a variety of animals as a volatile anaesthetic.

Permissible levels of trichloroethylene in the working environment have been established in various countries (Winell, 1975). The threshold limited value in the US is 535 mg/m^3 (100 ppm) and the maximum allowable concentration in the USSR is 10 mg/m^3.

The US Food and Drug Administration has approved the use of trichloroethylene as an extraction solvent only if residues do not exceed 25 mg/kg in decaffeinated ground coffee, 10 mg/kg in decaffeinated soluble (instant) coffee extract and 30 mg/kg total chlorinated solvents in spice oleoresins (US Code of Federal Regulations, 1975). The use of trichloroethylene for caffeine extraction has recently been discontinued in the US.

2.2 Occurrence

Air: Concentrations of trichloroethylene in air samples taken at 5 land stations ranged from 2-28 ng/m^3 (0.5-5 ppt)*, at 11 sea stations from 1-22 ng/m^3 (0.2-4 ppt) and over the northeast Atlantic Ocean from 5-11 ng/m^3 (1.2 ppt) (Murray & Riley, 1973). The reported concentration in the North Atlantic in October 1973 was less than 25 ng/m^3 (5 ppt) (Lovelock, 1974).

The background concentration of trichloroethylene in the atmosphere during June and July 1974 in Western Ireland was 80 ng/m^3 (15 ppt) (Lovelock, 1974). Typical concentrations at 8 locations in 5 US states in 1974 ranged from 970 ng/m^3 (180 ppt) in urban areas to less than 110 ng/m^3 (20 ppt) in rural areas (Lillian *et al.*, 1975). Less than 30 ng/m^3 (5 ppt) were found in air samples in rural Pullman, Washington, from December 1974 to February 1975 (Grimsrud & Rasmussen, 1975).

---

*ppt = parts per 10^{12}

It has been estimated that the concentration of trichloroethylene in the northern hemisphere is about 80 ng/m^3 (15 ppt), and that in the southern hemisphere, about 8 ng/m^3 (1.5 ppt) (Yung *et al.*, 1975).

Occupational: The number of US workers exposed to trichloroethylene has been estimated to be about 283 thousand (Lloyd *et al.*, 1975). Levels of 1076-43,000 mg/m^3 (200-8000 ppm) were found in a small American factory (Kleinfeld & Tabershaw, 1954).

Concentrations of vapour in a dial assembly workshop in a Japanese factory ranged from below 135 mg/m^3 (25 ppm) to over 538 mg/m^3 (100 ppm). Concentrations in the degreasing room were between 800 and 1350 mg/m^3 (150-250 ppm) (Takamatsu, 1962).

The concentration to which surgeons and nurses were exposed in operating-rooms varied from 1.6-554 mg/m^3 (0.3-103 ppm) (Corbett, 1973). About 5000 medical, dental and hospital personnel are routinely exposed to trichloroethylene.

Water: Analysis of water at a sewage treatment plant in Ohio in 1974 showed that the level of trichloroethylene was slightly enhanced by chlorination (Bellar *et al.*, 1974). In another study, trichloroethylene was found in the organic constituents of Mississippi river water (before and after treatment) and of commercial deionized charcoal-filtered water (Dowty *et al.*, 1975).

Food: Traces of trichloroethylene have been found in edible oils after extraction (Gracián & Martel, 1972). Levels of trichloroethylene in foodstuffs such as dairy products, meat, oils and fats, beverages and fruits and vegetables ranged from 0.02 µg/kg in wine to 60 µg/kg in packaged tea (McConnell *et al.*, 1975).

Human tissues: Quantities of trichloroethylene in post-mortem samples were from less than 1 to 32 µg/kg wet tissue (McConnell *et al.*, 1975).

2.3 Analysis

A review of the analysis and characteristics of trichloroethylene wastes in water-treatment plant sludge was made by Camisa (1975).

Gas chromatography with detection by flame-ionization was used for the determination of trichloroethylene in the atmosphere of workplaces (Herbolsheimer et al., 1972; White et al., 1970); the limit of detection was 5 mg/m^3 (1 ppm). Gas chromatography-mass spectrometry was used to analyse atmospheric samples (Grimsrud & Rasmussen, 1975) and drinking-water (Novak et al., 1973). Sewage and industrial waste waters were analysed using both gas chromatography with flame-ionization detection and infra-red spectroscopy (Ellison & Wallbank, 1973). Gas chromatography with detection by thermal conductivity was used in air samples (Grupinski, 1971). Several authors state that electron-capture detection is more sensitive than flame-ionization detection, but limits of detection are not given. Electron capture/gas chromatography has been used to detect trichloroethylene in spice oleoresins (Page & Kennedy, 1975).

3. Biological Data Relevant to the Evaluation of Carcinogenic Risk to Man

3.1 Carcinogenicity and related studies in animals

Oral administration

Mouse: Twenty-eight NLC mice (age not specified) were given oral doses by gavage of 0.1 ml of a 40% solution of trichloroethylene in oil twice weekly for an unspecified period. No liver lesions or hepatomas were observed. Administration of carbon tetrachloride or chloroform to the same strain of mice induced hepatomas (Rudali, 1967).

Gastric intubation of 2.4 or 1.2 g/kg bw trichloroethylene 5 times weekly in male B6C3F mice (age not specified) and of 1.8 or 0.9 g/kg bw in females induced hepatocellular carcinomas in 30/98 (30.6%) mice given the low dose and in 41/95 (43.2%) mice given the higher dose. Hepatocellular carcinomas occurred in 1/40 (2.5%) control mice (Lloyd et al., 1975).

Rat: Gastric intubation of either 1.0 or 0.5 g/kg bw of the compound in both sexes of Osborne-Mendel rats (age not specified), 5 times weekly for an unspecified period produced no hepatocellular carcinomas (Lloyd et al., 1975).

3.2 Other relevant biological data

(a) Experimental systems

The extensive literature on toxicity of trichloroethylene has been reviewed by Browning (1965), Lloyd et al. (1975), von Oettingen (1964) and Smith (1966).

The oral LD_{50}'s (causing death in 24 hours) were 3.2 g/kg bw for mice (Klaassen & Plaa, 1966) and 2.8 g/kg bw for dogs (Klaassen & Plaa, 1967). The maximum concentrations of vapour which produced no toxic effects after exposure for 7 hours daily on 5 days a week for 6 months were: rats and rabbits, 1076 mg/m³ (200 ppm); guinea-pigs, 538 mg/m³ (100 ppm); monkeys, 2052 mg/m³ (400 ppm) (Adams et al., 1951).

In 8 cats exposed to concentrations of 108 mg/m³ of air (20 ppm) for 1-1.5 hours per day for 4-6 months, centrilobular necrosis, nephritis, hypertrophy of lymphoid glands and splenomegaly were observed (Mosinger & Fiorentini, 1955). In mice, trichloroethylene caused less damage to the kidneys and liver than did carbon tetrachloride or chloroform (Klaassen & Plaa, 1966).

In rats and dogs, trichloroethylene is concentrated mostly in fat, brain, skeletal muscle, lung and liver (Barrett et al., 1939). Unchanged trichloroethylene was excreted via the lungs of exposed animals (Browning, 1965).

When ^{36}Cl-trichloroethylene was given by gavage to rats, 10-20% of the dose was excreted in the urine as 1-5% trichloroacetic acid and 10-15% trichloroethanol, 0-0.5% was excreted as trichloroethylene in the faeces and 72-85% as trichloroethylene in the expired air (Daniel, 1963). It is also metabolized to trichloroethanol and trichloroacetic acid in dogs (Barrett & Johnston, 1939; Butler, 1949). The suggestion (Powell, 1945) that formation of these metabolites implies rearrangement of the transient trichloroethylene oxide intermediate into chloral has been confirmed (a) by study of the rearrangement of the oxides belonging to a series of chlorinated ethylenes (Bonse et al., 1975), and (b) by the identification of chloral as a trichloroethylene metabolite in vitro (Byington & Leibman, 1965) and in vivo (Sconsetti et al., 1959).

Trichloroethylene turnover in rats was lowered by simultaneous administration of toluene (Ikeda, 1974).

A 2-hour treatment with 3.3 mM trichloroethylene in the presence of a metabolic activating microsomal system induced reverse mutations in *Escherichia coli* strain K12 (Greim *et al.*, 1975). Chloral hydrate, a metabolite of trichloroethylene is mutagenic in *Antirrhinum* (Barthelmess, 1956).

(b) Man

Death occurred in four workers exposed to concentrations of 1076-43,000 mg/m^3 (200-8000 ppm) trichloroethylene. A fifth death occurred due to accidental drinking of trichloroethylene (Kleinfeld & Tabershaw, 1954). Irritation of the lungs and gastrointestinal tract have been reported after industrial over-exposure (Browning, 1965). Chronic inhalation affects the central nervous system (Grandjean *et al.*, 1955) and may cause disturbance of protein metabolism (Guyotjeannin & Van Steenkiste, 1958).

Exposure of volunteers to 592 mg/m^3 (110 ppm) trichloroethylene for two 4-hour periods resulted in a statistically significant decrease in performance ability in the tachistoscopic apperception test, in the Wechsler memory scale, in a complex reaction time test and in a manual dexterity test (Salvini *et al.*, 1971).

In man, trichloroethylene is excreted as trichloroacetic acid (7-27%) (Powell, 1945) and trichloroethanol (about 20%) (Browning, 1965; Kimmerle & Eben, 1973). Trichloroacetic acid was found in the urine 2-3 times more often and trichloroethanol 2-3 times less often in women than in men in the first 24 hours after exposure (Nomiyama & Nomiyama, 1971). A relatively high retention of trichloroethylene occurred after inhalation of 1250-1900 mg/m^3 (250-380 ppm) for 2.7 hours (33% in men, 37% in women). It was eliminated *via* the lung less rapidly in women (17%) than in men (22%) (Nomiyama & Nomiyama, 1974).

3.3 Observations in man

No data were available to the Working Group.

4. Comments on Data Reported and Evaluation

4.1 Animal data

According to a preliminary report, trichloroethylene induced liver-cell carcinomas in mice but not in rats after its oral administration.

4.2 Human data

No case reports or epidemiological studies were available to the Working Group.

5. References

Adams, E.M., Spencer, H.C., Rowe, V.K., McCollister, D.D. & Irish, D.D. (1951) Vapor toxicity of trichloroethylene determined by experiments on laboratory animals. *A.M.A. industr. Hyg. occup. Med.*, 4, 469-481

Anon. (1972) Solvent growth rates scrambled by strong environmental signals: hydrocarbons, ketones hurting. *Chemical Marketing Reporter*, May 8, pp. 3, 47

Barrett, H.M. & Johnston, J.H. (1939) The fate of trichloroethylene in the organism. *J. biol. Chem.*, 127, 765-770

Barrett, H.M., Cunningham, J.G. & Johnston, J.H. (1939) A study of the fate in the organism of some chlorinated hydrocarbons. *J. industr. Hyg. Toxicol.*, 21, 479-490

Barthelmess, A. (1956) Mutagene Arzneimittel. *Arzneimittelforsch.*, 6, 157-168

Bellar, T.A., Lichtenberg, J.J. & Kroner, R.C. (1974) The occurrence of organohalides in chlorinated drinking water. *J. Amer. Water Works Ass.*, 66, 703-706

Bonse, G., Urban, T., Reichert, D. & Henschler, D. (1975) Chemical reactivity, metabolic oxirane formation and biological reactivity of chlorinated ethylenes in the isolated perfused rat liver preparation. *Biochem. Pharmacol.*, 24, 1829-1834

Browning, E. (1965) *Toxicity and Metabolism of Industrial Solvents*, Amsterdam, Elsevier, pp. 189-212

Butler, T.C. (1949) Metabolic transformations of trichloroethylene. *J. Pharmacol. exp. Ther.*, 97, 84-92

Byington, K.H. & Leibman, K.C. (1965) Metabolism of trichloroethylene by liver microsomes. II. Identification of the reaction product as chloral hydrate. *Molec. Pharmacol.*, 1, 247-254

Camisa, A.G. (1975) Analysis and characteristics of trichloroethylene wastes. *J. Water Poll. Control Fed.*, 47, 1021-1031

Copelin, H.B. (1954) Stabilization of chlorinated hydrocarbons. *US Patent* 2,797,250, May 13 to E.I. Du Pont de Nemours & Co

Corbett, T.H. (1973) Retention of anesthetic agents following occupational exposure. *Anesth. Analg. Curr. Res.*, 52, 614-618

Daniel, J.W. (1963) The metabolism of Cl-labelled trichloroethylene and tetrachloroethylene in the rat. *Biochem. Pharmacol.*, 12, 795-802

Dowty, B.J., Carlisle, D.R. & Laseter, J.L. (1975) New Orleans drinking water sources tested by gas chromatography-mass spectrometry. Occurrence and origin of aromatics and halogenated aliphatic hydrocarbons. Environm. Sci. Technol., 9, 762-765

Ellison, W.K. & Wallbank, T.E. (1973) Solvents in sewage and industrial waste waters: identification and determination. Wat. Poll. Contr., 73, 656-672

Gracián, J. & Martel, J. (1972) Determinación de residuos de disolventes en aceites refinados comestibles. I. Grasa Aceites (Seville), 23, 1-6

Grandjean, E., Münchinger, R., Turrian, V., Haas, P.A., Knoepfel, H.K. & Rosenmund, H. (1955) Investigations into the effects of exposure to trichloroethylene in mechanical engineering. Brit. J. industr. Med., 12, 131-142

Grasselli, J.G., ed. (1973) Atlas of Spectral Data and Physical Constants for Organic Compounds, Cleveland, Ohio, Chemical Rubber Co., p. B-520

Greim, H., Bonse, G., Radwan, Z., Reichert, D. & Henschler, D. (1975) Mutagenicity *in vitro* and potential carcinogenicity of chlorinated ethylenes as a function of metabolic oxirane formation. Biochem. Pharmacol., 24, 2013-2017

Grimsrud, E.P. & Rasmussen, R.A. (1975) Survey and analysis of halocarbons in the atmosphere by gas chromatography-mass spectrometry. Atmosph. Environm., 9, 1014-1017

Grupinski, L. (1971) Determination of the concentrations of chlorinated hydrocarbons in air by means of gas chromatography. Staub-Reinhalt. Luft, 31, 3-7

Guyotjeannin, C. & van Steenkiste, J. (1958) Action du trichloréthylène sur les protéines et les lipides sériques. Etude chez 18 ouvriers travaillant en atmosphère polluée. Arch. Malad. prof., 19, 489-494

Hardie, D.W.F. (1964) Chlorocarbons and chlorohydrocarbons. Trichloroethylene. In: Kirk, R.E. & Othmer, D.F., eds, Encyclopedia of Chemical Technology, 2nd ed., Vol. 5, New York, John Wiley and Sons, pp. 183-195

Hawley, G.G., ed. (1971) Condensed Chemical Dictionary, 8th ed., New York, Van Nostrand-Reinhold, pp. 886-887

Herbolsheimer, R., Funk, L. & Drasche, H. (1972) Usability of activated carbon as adsorbant for the determination of trichloroethylene in the air. Staub-Reinhalt. Luft, 32, 31-33

Ikeda, M. (1974) Reciprocal metabolic inhibition of toluene and trichloroethylene *in vivo* and *in vitro*. Int. Arch. Arbeitsmed., 33, 125-130

Irish, D. (1962) Trichloroethylene. In: Patty, F.A., ed., Industrial Hygiene and Toxicology, 2nd ed., Vol. II, New York, Interscience, pp. 1309-1313

Jordan, T.E. (1954) Vapor Pressure of Organic Compounds, New York, Interscience, p. 48

Kimmerle, G. & Eben, A. (1973) Metabolism, excretion and toxicology of trichloroethylene after inhalation. Arch. Toxikol., 30, 127-138

Klaassen, C.D. & Plaa, G.L. (1966) Relative effects of various chlorinated hydrocarbons on liver and kidney function in mice. Toxicol. appl. Pharmacol., 9, 139-151

Klaassen, C.D. & Plaa, G.L. (1967) Relative effects of various chlorinated hydrocarbons on liver and kidney function in dogs. Toxicol. appl. Pharmacol., 10, 119-131

Kleinfeld, M. & Tabershaw, I. (1954) Trichloroethylene toxicity. Report of five fatal cases. A.M.A. Arch. industr. Hyg., 10, 134-141

Lillian, D., Singh, H., Appleby, A., Lobban, L., Arnts, R., Gumpert, R., Hague, R., Toomey, J., Kazazis, J., Antell, M., Hansen, D. & Scott, B. (1975) Atmospheric fates of halogenated compounds. Environm. Sci. Technol., 9, 1042-1048

Lloyd, J.W., Moore, R.M., Jr & Breslin, P. (1975) Background information on trichloroethylene. J. occup. Med., 17, 603-605

Lovelock, J.E. (1974) Atmospheric halocarbons and stratospheric ozone. Nature (Lond.), 252, 292-294

McConnell, G., Ferguson, D.M. & Pearson, C.R. (1975) Chlorinated hydrocarbons and the environment. Endeavour, 34, 13-18

Mosinger, M. & Fiorentini, H. (1955) Réactions hépatiques, rénales, ganglionnaires et spléniques dans l'intoxication expérimentale par le trichloréthylène chez le chat. C.R. Soc. Biol. (Paris), 149, 150-152

Murray, A.J. & Riley, J.R. (1973) Occurrence of some chlorinated aliphatic hydrocarbons in the environment. Nature (Lond.), 242, 37-38

Nomiyama, K. & Nomiyama, H. (1971) Metabolism of trichloroethylene in human. Int. Arch. Arbeitsmed., 28, 37-48

Nomiyama, K. & Nomiyama, H. (1974) Respiratory retention, uptake and excretion of organic solvents in man. Benzene, toluene, n-hexane, trichloroethylene, acetone, ethyl acetate and ethyl alcohol. Int. Arch. Arbeitsmed., 32, 75-83

Novak, J., Zluticky, J., Kubelka, V. & Mostecky, J. (1973) Analysis of organic constituents present in drinking water. J. Chromat., 76, 45-50 von Oettingen, W.F. (1964) The Halogenated Hydrocarbons of Industrial and Toxicological Importance, Amsterdam, Elsevier, pp. 240-271

Page, B.D. & Kennedy, B.P.C. (1975) Determination of methylene chloride, ethylene dichloride and trichloroethylene as solvent residues in spice oleoresins, using vacuum distillation and electron capture gas chromatography. J. Ass. off. Analyt. Chem., 58, 1062-1068

Powell, J.F. (1945) Trichloroethylene: absorption, elimination and metabolism. Brit. J. industr. Med., 2, 142-145

Rudali, G. (1967) A propos de l'activité oncogène de quelques hydrocarbures halogénés utilisés en thérapeutique. UICC Monograph, 7, 138-143

Salvini, M., Binaschi, S. & Riva, M. (1971) Evaluation of the psychophysiological functions in humans exposed to trichloroethylene. Brit. J. industr. Med., 28, 293-295

Scansetti, G., Rubino, G.F. & Trompeo, G. (1959) Studio sull'intossicazione cronica da trielina. III. Metabolismo del trichloroetilene. Med. lavoro, 50, 743-754

Smith, G.F. (1966) Trichloroethylene: a review. Brit. J. industr. Med., 23, 249-262

Starks, F.W. (1956) Stabilization of chlorinated hydrocarbons. US Patent 2,818,446, October 25, to E.I. Du Pont de Nemours & Co.

Takamatsu, M. (1962) Health hazards in workers exposed to trichloroethylene vapor. II. Exposure to trichloroethylene during degreasing operation in a communicating machine factory. Kumamoto med. J., 15, 43-54

US Code of Federal Regulations (1975) Trichloroethylene, Food and Drugs, Title 21, part 121.1041, Washington DC, US Government Printing Office, pp. 428-429

US Department of Commerce (1975a) US Exports, Bureau of the Census, FT 410/December 1974, Washington DC, US Government Printing Office, p. 86

US Department of Commerce (1975b) US General Imports, Bureau of the Census, FT 135/December 1974, Washington DC, US Government Printing Office, p. 2-139

US International Trade Commission (1975a) Preliminary Report on US Production of Selected Synthetic Organic Chemicals, Preliminary Totals, 1974, S.O.C. Series C/P-75-1, May 16, Washington DC, US Government Printing Office, p. 2

US International Trade Commission (1975b) Preliminary Report on US Production of Selected Synthetic Organic Chemicals, August, September and Cumulative Totals, 1975, S.O.C. Series C/P-75-9, November 5, Washington DC, US Government Printing Office, p. 3

US Tariff Commission (1972) Synthetic Organic Chemicals, US Production and Sales, 1970, TC Publication 479, Washington DC, US Government Printing Office, pp. 215, 241

Weast, R.C., ed. (1975) Handbook of Chemistry and Physics, 56th ed., Cleveland, Ohio, Chemical Rubber Co., p. C-292

White, L.D., Taylor, D.G., Mauer, P.A. & Kupel, R.E. (1970) A convenient optimized method for the analysis of selected solvent vapors in the industrial atmosphere. Amer. industr. Hyg. Ass. J., 31, 225-232

Winell, M.A. (1975) An international comparison of hygienic standards for chemicals in the work environment. Ambio, 4, 34-36

Yung, Y.L., McElroy, M.B. & Wofsy, S.C. (1975) Atmospheric halocarbons: a discussion with emphasis on chloroform. Geophys. Res. Lett., 2, 397-399

4-VINYLCYCLOHEXENE*

1. Chemical and Physical Data

1.1 Synonyms and trade names

Chem. Abstr. Reg. Serial No.: 100-40-3

Chem. Abstr. Name: 4-Ethenyl-1-cyclohexene

Cyclohexenylethylene; 1-ethenylcyclohexene; 1,2,3,4-tetrahydrostyrene; 4-vinyl-1-cyclohexene; 4-vinylcyclohexene-1; 1-vinylcyclohexene-3

1.2 Chemical formula and molecular weight

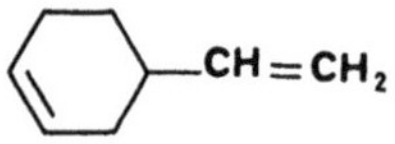

C_8H_{12} Mol. wt: 108.2

1.3 Chemical and physical properties

From Weast (1975), unless otherwise specified

(a) Description: Liquid

(b) Boiling-point: 145°C at 760 mm; 50-52°C at 22 mm

(c) Density: d_4^{15} 0.8623

(d) Refractive index: n_D^{20} 1.4915

(e) Spectroscopy data: λ_{max} 230; E_1^1 = 1935 (in ethanol) (Hawley, 1971); ultra-violet spectrum is given by Grasselli (1973); mass spectrum is given by Brittain (1969)

(f) Solubility: Immiscible with water; miscible with ether, benzene and methanol

---

*Considered by the Working Group, February 1976

(g) _Stability_: Oxidizes in air to form the hydroperoxide

1.4 Technical products and impurities

4-Vinylcyclohexene is available as a technical grade of 95% purity and as a grade for laboratory research with 99% purity. Since it is prepared by dimerization of butadiene, the most likely contaminant is cyclooctadiene (Hawley, 1971; Sittig, 1968); since it is easily oxidized in air, the hydroperoxide is also a contaminant. About 50 mg/kg oxidation inhibitor are usually present (Vollmar, 1971).

2. Production, Use, Occurrence and Analysis

For important background information on this section, see preamble, p. 19

2.1 Production and use

4-Vinylcyclohexene can be prepared by the dimerization of butadiene at 425°C and 13 atm using a silicon-carbide catalyst, or at 100-150°C and 40-1000 atm using copper or chromium salts of naphthenic or resin acids. It is formed on prolonged storage of butadiene (Kirshenbaum & Cahn, 1964) and is believed to be produced commercially as a by-product of one method of butadiene manufacture. Although 4-vinylcyclohexene is probably made and consumed as an intermediate by several US chemical manufacturers, only one company has reported production.

4-Vinylclohexene is used as an intermediate for the production of vinylcyclohexene dioxide, which is used as a reactive diluent in epoxy resins. Although 4-vinylcyclohexene may also have been used at low levels as a co-monomer in the polymerization of other monomers (e.g., styrene) and for halogenation to polyhalogenated derivatives used as flame retardants, no evidence was found that it is now being used in such applications.

2.2 Occurrence

Concentrations of 4-vinylcyclohexene at its site of manufacture have averaged 1.2-2.4 g/m^3 and have on occasion reached 3 g/m^3 (Bykov, 1968).

2.3 Analysis

Gas chromatography was used by Carson & Lege (1974) to determine the quantity of 4-vinylcyclohexene formed from butadiene by its dimerization in the gas chromatograph.

3. Biological Data Relevant to the Evaluation of Carcinogenic Risk to Man

3.1 Carcinogenicity and related studies in animals

Skin application

Mouse: of 30 8-week old Swiss ICR/Ha male mice treated with 45 mg 4-vinylcyclohexene in 0.1 ml of a 50% solution in benzene on the clipped dorsal skin thrice weekly for life, 6 developed skin tumours; one of these had a squamous-cell carcinoma; the median survival time was 375 days. Of 150 control mice painted with benzene alone, 10 developed skin papillomas and 1 a carcinoma. The compound was purified by removing autoxidation products with ferrous sulphate, but it is possible that it contained a minute amount of the hydroperoxide formed by autoxidation (Van Duuren *et al.*, 1963) [The increased tumour incidence is significant: $P<0.02$].

When 'oxygen-free material' (0.1 ml of a 10% solution in benzene) was applied thrice weekly for life to 30 male Swiss ICR/Ha mice, the median survival time was 565 days, and no carcinogenic effect was observed (Van Duuren, 1965).

3.2 Other relevant biological data

The single oral LD_{50} of 4-vinylcyclohexene in rats is 2.6 g/kg bw, and the percutaneous LD_{50} in rabbits is 17 g/kg bw (Smyth *et al.*, 1969). The inhalation LD_{50}'s in mice and rats are 27 and 47 g/m^3, respectively. When 1 g/m^3 was administered by inhalation for 6 hours/day over 4 months, 4-vinylcyclohexene inhibited weight increase and caused leucocytosis, leucopenia and impairment of haemodynamics in rats and mice (Bykov, 1968).

(b) Man

Keratitis, rhinitis, headache, hypotonia, leucopenia, neutrophilia, lymphocytosis and impairment of pigment and carbohydrate metabolism have been noted in workers exposed to 4-vinylcyclohexene (Bykov, 1968).

3.3 Observations in man

No data were available to the Working Group.

4. Comments on Data Reported and Evaluation

4.1 Animal data

Vinylcyclohexene has been tested only in mice by skin application. The data do not allow an evaluation.

4.2 Human data

No case reports or epidemiological studies were available to the Working Group.

5. References

Brittain, E.F.H., Wells, C.H.J. & Parsley, H.M. (1969) Mass spectra of isomers. III. Cyclo-octadiene and derivatives of cyclobutane and cyclohexene of molecular formula C_8H_{12}. J. chem. Soc., B, 503-505

Bykov, L.A. (1968) Maximum permissible concentration of vinylcyclohexene in the air of industrial buildings. In: Proceedings of a Conference on the Toxicology and Hygiene of Petrochemical Industrial Products, Moscow, pp. 32-34

Carson, J.W. & Lege, G.J. (1974) Butadiene dimer formation in chromatograph vaporizers. J. chromat. Sci., 12, 49-50

Grasselli, J.S. (1973) Atlas of Spectral and Physical Constants for Organic Compounds, Cleveland, Ohio, Chemical Rubber Co., p. B-456

Hawley, G.G., ed. (1971) The Condensed Chemical Dictionary, 8th ed., New York, Van Nostrand-Reinhold, p. 927

Kirshenbaum, I. & Cahn, R.P. (1964) Butadiene. In: Kirk, R.E. & Othmer, D.F., eds, Encyclopedia of Chemical Technology, 2nd ed., Vol. 3, New York, John Wiley and Sons, pp. 786-787

Sittig, M. (1968) Diolefins - Manufacture and Derivatives, Chemical Process Review No. 16, Parkridge, NY, Noyes Development Corp.

Smyth, H.F., Jr, Carpenter, C.P., Weil, C.S., Pozzani, U.C., Striegel, J.A. & Nycum, J.S. (1969) Range-finding toxicity data: list VII. Amer. industr. Hyg. Ass. J., 30, 470-476

Van Duuren, B.L. (1965) Carcinogenic epoxides, lactones and hydroperoxides. In: Wogan, G.N., ed., Mycotoxins in Foodstuffs, Cambridge, Massachusetts Institute of Technology Press, pp. 275-285

Van Duuren, B.L., Nelson, N., Orris, L., Palmes, E.D. & Schmitt, F.L. (1963) Carcinogenicity of epoxides, lactones and peroxy compounds. J. nat. Cancer Inst., 31, 41-55

Vollmar, R.C. (1971) Dienes. In: Encyclopedia of Industrial Chemical Analysis, Vol. 2, New York, Interscience, pp. 512-514

Weast, R.C., ed. (1975) Handbook of Chemistry and Physics, 56th ed., Cleveland, Ohio, Chemical Rubber Co., p. C-259

GENERAL CONSIDERATIONS ON VOLATILE ANAESTHETICS

GENERAL CONSIDERATIONS ON VOLATILE ANAESTHETICS*

Inhalational anaesthesia was discovered in 1842. Since that time a number of chemical compounds have been used as anaesthetics; the most widely used agents and the year in which each was introduced as an anaesthetic are as follows:

Anaesthetic	Chem. Abstr. Reg. Serial No.	Year of introduction as anaesthetic
Diethyl ether	60-29-7	1842
Nitrous oxide	10024-97-2	1845
Chloroform	67-66-3	1847
Cyclopropane	75-19-4	1933
Trichloroethylene	79-01-6	1934
Fluroxene	406-90-6	1954
Halothane	151-67-7	1956
Methoxyflurane	76-38-0	1960
Enflurane	13838-16-9	1974
Isoflurane	26675-46-7	-

Administered in conjunction with other anaesthetics, nitrous oxide is the most commonly used volatile anaesthetic. Of the halogenated compounds, halothane is the most frequently used, followed by enflurane, methoxyflurane and trichloroethylene. Chloroform, cyclopropane and fluroxene are no longer widely used as anaesthetics. Diethyl ether is still used in various countries.

Anaesthetics are administered approximately twenty million times each year to patients in the twenty-five thousand operating rooms throughout the US. Approximately fifty thousand operating room personnel are exposed daily to low concentrations of anaesthetic gases which occur in operating rooms during the administration of inhalational anaesthesia. Surgeons are not

---

*Considered by the Working Group, February 1976

included in this estimate, since they usually do not operate every day and are thus less exposed. The following table lists the numbers of operating-room workers in the US by professional group (Cohen et al., 1974):

Professional Group	Membership (1973)
American Society of Anesthesiologists	11,192
American Association of Nurse-anesthetists	14,594
Associations of Operating Room Nurses and Technicians (combined)	23,799

Some veterinarians and an unknown number of workers engaged in the production of the various anaesthetic agents are exposed to these chemicals in their working environments.

Inhalational anaesthetics are usually administered *via* machines which mix the appropriate gases and vapours at the desired concentrations. A high-flow, semi-closed rebreathing system with a carbon dioxide absorber is most commonly used. Flow rates in high-flow systems are usually maintained at 5-6 litres of gas per minute. The patient uses less than 0.5 litre per minute, the excess gases escaping into the operating room through a 'pop-off' valve located on the anaesthesia machine. This valve is usually located within 0.5-1 metre of the person administering the anaesthetic.

A wide range of concentrations are delivered to patients, depending on the anaesthetic used. The potent halogenated hydrocarbons and halogenated ethers are generally administered at levels of 0.2-2% for maintenance of anaesthesia, while the less potent nitrous oxide is usually delivered in concentrations ranging from 50-67%.

In a study of the concentrations of anaesthetics occurring in operating-rooms, 392 mg/m^3 (49 ppm) halothane and 526 mg/m^3 (428 ppm) nitrous oxide were found (Linde & Bruce, 1969). Askrog & Petersen (1970) found average concentrations of 680 mg/m^3 (85 ppm) halothane and 8600 mg/m^3 (7000 ppm) nitrous oxide in the inhalation zone of anaesthetists when a non-rebreathing system was used. The ranges of concentrations of several anaesthetic agents in the operating-room environment under routine working conditions are as follows (Corbett, 1973, 1976):

Ranges of concentrations of anaesthetic agents
found in the operating-room environment

Agent	Near anaesthetist		Near surgeon	
	mg/m^3	ppm	mg/m^3	ppm
Nitrous oxide	406–11,900	330–9700	380–675	310–550
Halothane	8–208	1–26	8–16	1–2
Methoxyflurane	13.4–67	2–10	6.7–13.4	1–2
Trichloroethylene	5.5–550	1–103	1.6–8	0.3–1.5
Enflurane	37.5–345	5–46	7.5–60	1–8

The chemistry, absorption, distribution and metabolism of inhalational anaesthetics have been reviewed (Cohen, 1971; Wylie & Churchill-Davidson, 1972). Collins (1966) and Wylie & Churchill-Davidson (1972) have outlined several theories of the mechanism of action by which these chemicals produce anaesthesia.

Hepatotoxicity has been observed in patients treated with volatile anaesthetics (Subcommittee on the National Halothane Study, 1966). Cases of hepatic dysfunction attributed to chronic inhalation of low concentrations of halothane during occupational or other exposure have been reported; in two of these cases exacerbation of liver disease has been related to re-exposure to halothane (Belfrage et al., 1966; Klatskin & Kimberg, 1969).

Toxic nephropathy has been observed in patients following anaesthesia induced with methoxyflurane. The effects include polyuria with negative fluid balance and raised serum sodium, uric acid, creatinine and urea. The effects are not due to deficiency of anti-diuretic hormone (Crandell et al., 1966). The damage is generally reversible but is occasionally permanent and lethal. The effects are probably due to direct toxic action of the fluoride and oxalate metabolites on the kidney (Hollenberg et al., 1972; Panner et al., 1970). The renal toxicity of anaesthetics has been reviewed by Mazze & Cousins (1973).

Significantly impaired psychophysiological performance has been demonstrated in volunteers exposed for 4 hours to 120 mg/m^3 (15 ppm) halothane plus 615 mg/m^3 (500 ppm) nitrous oxide; a lesser impairment in performance followed exposure to 112 mg/m³ (15 ppm) enflurane plus 615 mg/m³ (500 ppm) nitrous oxide (Bruce & Bach, 1975; Bruce *et al.*, 1974).

After i.p. injection of ^{14}C-labelled chloroform and halothane to mice, radioactivity was bound preferentially to endoplasmic protein and lipid fractions in the liver. *In vitro*, in the presence of rabbit liver microsomes, oxygen and NADPH, covalent binding to protein fractions was also observed (Uehleke *et al.*, 1976).

The embryotoxic and teratogenic effects of anaesthetic concentrations of inhalational anaesthetics in animals have been well documented (Basford & Fink, 1968; Fink *et al.*, 1967; Smith *et al.*, 1965).

Rats exposed prenatally by administration to the dams of 80 mg/m³ (10 ppm) halothane for 8 hours per day on 5 days a week and postnatally up to 60 days after birth to the same concentration had later impairments in learning ability. Reduced learning ability was correlated with persistent synaptic malformation in the cerebral cortex. Other changes in the neurons noted in young adult rats exposed to 80 mg/m³ (10 ppm) halothane for 8 hours per day on 5 days a week for 8 weeks included destruction of the rough-surfaced endoplasmic reticulum, dilatation of the Golgi complex and focal cytoplasmic vacuolation (Quimby *et al.*, 1975). Offspring of rats exposed to 80 mg/m³ (10 ppm) halothane for 8 hours per day on 5 days a week throughout pregnancy had ultrastructural changes in the liver within 24 hours of birth. These changes included myelin figures and large areas of focal cytoplasmic degradation in many hepatocytes; accumulation of lipids within hepatocytes and leucocytic infiltration were noted in many cases. Focal necrosis was observed in more than 50% of tissue samples (Chang *et al.*, 1975).

Halothane inhibits phagocytosis in mice, rabbits and humans. *In vivo* studies in rodents have revealed a significant time-dependent reduction in splenic antibody-producing cells after 2 hours' exposure to 1% halothane and after 4 hours' exposure to 0.5% halothane. In rats, recovery of normal antibody-forming capacity did not occur until 72 hours after the end of anaesthesia. Changes in lymphocyte function were reflected in a decrease in antibody titre and complement fixation which did not occur until 24-48 hours after anaesthesia. The immunosuppressive effects of volatile anaesthetics in animals and man have been reviewed (Bruce & Wingard, 1971).

Nitrous oxide had different effects in various strains of rats on leucocyte counts and DNA/RNA ratios of thymus tissue (Green, 1968). Bone-marrow depression was observed in humans exposed for 4 days to high concentrations of nitrous oxide in the treatment of tetanus (Lassen et al., 1956).

Mutagenicity tests with halothane and chloroform in the presence of a liver activation system were negative with *Salmonella typhimurium* strains TA 1535 and TA 1538 and with *Escherischia coli* strain K-12 (Uehleke et al., 1976).

Carcinogenicity bioassays of volatile anaesthetics are lacking, although tests on trichloroethylene (see p.263) and isoflurane have been conducted. The latter compound produced a significant increase in the incidence of liver-cell tumours (hepatomas) in male mice exposed pre- and postnatally (Corbett, 1976). A carcinogenicity bioassay of halothane by inhalation is currently being carried out in Swiss/SWR mice (Corbett - USVA Hospital, Ann Arbor, Michigan, USA).

Epidemiological surveys of occupationally exposed populations have examined possible carcinogenic, teratogenic and mutagenic effects of chronic exposure to the operating-room environment.

In one study, a high rate of miscarriages (18/31) was observed among pregnant anaesthetists (Vaisman, 1967); and in another study, pregnancies among anaesthetists and nurses in anaesthetic departments ended in spontaneous abortion or premature delivery about twice as often (20% compared to 10%) as among unexposed women (Askrog & Harvald, 1970). In a third study, female anaesthetists were found to have a higher frequency of involuntary infertility (12% *versus* 6%) and spontaneous abortion (18.3% *versus* 14.7%) than unexposed women (Knill-Jones et al., 1972).

Birth defects occurred more frequently among children whose mothers worked in operating theatres during pregnancy than among children whose mothers did not (Corbett et al., 1974).

A national study performed in the US reported that women chronically exposed to the operating-room environment have increased risks of cancer, diseases of the liver and kidney, spontaneous abortion and congenital anomalies in their children. An increased incidence of congenital anomalies in children born to wives of male operating-room personnel was also noted (Cohen *et al.*, 1974).

A survey was carried out to determine the incidence of malignancy in 621 female nurse-anaesthetists in Michigan. A total of 33 malignancies, including malignant thymoma, leiomyosarcoma, hepatocellular carcinoma and carcinoma of the pancreas, were reported in 31 anaesthetists. Excluding skin cancers, the expected incidence, adjusted for age distribution on the basis of statistics from the Connecticut Tumor Registry, is 403/100,000 per annum. The adjusted incidence in Michigan nurse-anaesthetists is 1,333/100,000 per annum (P<0.035) (Corbett *et al.*, 1973). The incidence of cancer among offspring born to nurse-anaesthetists was also studied in this survey. Three neoplasms occurred in two of 434 children born to anaesthetists who worked during the pregnancy (a neuroblastoma and a carcinoma of the thyroid in one and a carcinoma of the parotid in the other), and one neoplasm (leukaemia) was reported among the 261 children born to anaesthetists who did not work during the pregnancy (Corbett *et al.*, 1974).

Available studies indicate that working in the operating-room environment is associated with an increased risk of cancer, teratogenic effects and, possibly, mutagenic effects, but it is not possible at the present time to determine which particular factors are responsible. Further epidemiological and laboratory studies are necessary.

5. References

Askrog, V. & Harvald, B. (1970) Teratogen effeck af inhalations-anaestetika. Nord. Med., 83, 498-500

Askrog, V. & Petersen, R. (1970) Forurening af operationsstuer med luftformige anaestetika og rontgenbestråling. Nord. Med., 83, 501-504

Basford, A. & Fink, B.R. (1968) The teratogenicity of halothane in the rat. Anesthesiology, 29, 1167-1173

Belfrage, S., Ahlgren, I. & Axelson, S. (1966) Halothane hepatitis in an anaesthetist. Lancet, ii, 1466-1467

Bruce, D.L. & Bach, M.J. (1975) Psychological studies of human performance as affected by traces of enflurane and nitrous oxide. Anesthesiology, 42, 194-196

Bruce, D.L. & Wingard, D.W. (1971) Anesthesia and the immune response. Anesthesiology, 24, 271-292

Bruce, D.L., Bach, M.J. & Arbit, J. (1974) Trace anesthetic effects on perceptual, cognitive, and motor skills. Anesthesiology, 40, 453-458

Chang, L.W., Lee, Y.K., Dudley, A.W., Jr & Katz, J. (1975) Ultrastructural evidence of the hepatotoxic effect of halothane in rats following *in utero* exposure. Canad. Anaesth. Soc. J., 22, 330-338

Cohen, E. (1971) Metabolism of the volatile anaesthetics. Anesthesiology, 35, 193-202

Cohen, E.N., Brown, B.W., Bruce, D.L., Cascorbi, H.F., Corbett, T.H., Jones, T.W. & Whitcher, C.H. (1974) Occupational disease among operating room personnel: a national survey. Report of an *ad hoc* committee on the effect of trace anesthetics on the health of operating room personnel, American Society of Anesthesiologists. Anesthesiology, 41, 321-340

Collins, V. (1966) Principles of Anesthesiology, Philadelphia, Lea & Febiger, pp. 921-932

Corbett, T.H. (1973) Retention of anesthetic agents following occupational exposure. Anesth. Analg. Curr. Res., 52, 614-618

Corbett, T.H. (1976) Cancer and congenital anomalies associated with anesthetics. Proc. nat. Acad. Sci. (Wash.) (in press)

Corbett, T.H., Cornell, R.G., Lieding, K. & Endres, J.L. (1973) Incidence of cancer among Michigan nurse-anesthetists. Anesthesiology, 38, 260-263

Corbett, T.H., Cornell, R.G., Endres, J.L. & Lieding, K. (1974) Birth defects among children of nurse-anesthetists. Anesthesiology, 41, 341-344

Crandell, W.B., Pappas, S.G. & Macdonald, A. (1966) Nephrotoxicity associated with methoxyflurane anesthesia. Anesthesiology, 27, 591-607

Fink, B.R., Shepard, T.H. & Blandau, R.J. (1967) Teratogenic activity of nitrous oxide. Nature (Lond.), 214, 146-148

Green, C.D. (1968) The effect of N_2O on RNA and DNA content of rat bone marrow and thymus. In: Fink, B.R., ed., Toxicity of Anesthetics, Baltimore, Williams & Wilkins, pp. 114-122

Hollenberg, N.K., McDonald, F.D., Cotran, R., Galvanek, E.G., Warhol, M., Vandam, L.D. & Merill, J.P. (1972) Irreversible acute oliguric renal failure : a complication of methoxyflurane anaesthesia. New Engl. J. Med., 286, 877-879

Knill-Jones, R.P., Moir, D.D., Rodrigues, L.V. & Spence, A.A. (1972) Anaesthetic practice and pregnancy. Lancet, ii, 1326-1328

Klatskin, G. & Kimberg, D.V. (1969) Recurrent hepatitis attributable to halothane sensitization in an anesthetist. New Engl. J. Med., 280, 515-522

Lassen, H.C.A., Henriksen, E.K., Neukirch, F. & Kristensen, H.S. (1956) Treatment of tetanus: severe bone-marrow depression after prolonged nitrous-oxide anaesthesia. Lancet, i, 527-530

Linde, H.W. & Bruce, D.L. (1969) Occupational exposure of anesthesiologists to halothane, N_2O and radiation. Anesthesiology, 30, 363-368

Mazze, R.I. & Cousins, M.J. (1973) Renal toxicity of anaesthetics : with specific reference to the nephrotoxicity of methoxyflurane. Canad. Anaesth. Soc. J., 20, 64-80

Panner, B.J., Freeman, R.B., Roth-Moyo, L.A. & Markowitch, W., Jr (1970) Toxicity following methoxyflurane anesthesia. I. Clinical and pathological observations in two fatal cases. J. Amer. med. Ass., 214, 86-90

Quimby, K., Katz, J. & Bowman, R. (1975) Behavioural consequences in rats from chronic exposure to 10 ppm halothane during early development. Anesth. Analg. Curr. Res., 54, 628-633

Smith, B.E., Gaub, M.L. & Moya, F. (1965) Investigation into the teratogenic effects of anesthetic agents. The fluorinated agents. Anesthesiology, 26, 260-261

Subcommittee on the National Halothane Study of the Committee on Anesthesia, National Academy of Sciences - National Research Council (1966) Summary of the national halothane study, possible association between halothane and postoperative hepatic necrosis. J. Amer. med. Ass., 197, 775-778

Uehleke, H., Greim, H., Krämer, M. & Werner, T. (1976) Covalent binding of haloalkanes to liver constituents, but absence of mutagenicity on bacteria in a metabolizing test system. Mutation Res., 38, 114

Vaisman, A.I. (1967) Working conditions in surgery and their effect on the health of anesthesiologists. Eksp. Khir. Anesteziol., 3, 44-49

Wylie, W. & Churchill-Davidson, H.C. (1972) Practice of Anaesthesia, 3rd ed., Chicago, Ill., Year Book Medical Pubs, Inc., pp. 266-280, 313-345, 623-625

SUPPLEMENTARY CORRIGENDA TO VOLUMES 1 - 10

A corrigenda covering Volumes 1 - 6 appeared in Volume 7, others appeared in Volumes 8 and 10. The present one covers further errors which have since been brought to our attention.

Volume 1

p. 111   para 4   line 4   *replace* 0.04 µg/litre *by* 0.04 g/litre

Volume 7

p. 157   4.1   lines 4-5   *replace* renal and hepatic *by* renal, hepatic and

p. 215   (b)   line 10   *replace* Ten occupations *by* Nine occupations
              line 12   *replace* 14 controls *by* 13 controls
              line 16   *replace* ten occupations *by* nine occupations

Volume 8

p. 68   4   *Add* [1] *to title of section*
            Add footnote [1]See also the section "Animal Data in Relation to the Evaluation of Risk to Man" in the introduction to this volume, p. 15

Volume 10

p. 188   line 1   *insert* not *between* was *and* greater

CUMULATIVE INDEX TO IARC MONOGRAPHS ON THE EVALUATION
OF CARCINOGENIC RISK OF CHEMICALS TO MAN

Numbers underlined indicate volume, and numbers in italics indicate page. References to corrigenda are given in parentheses.

Acetamide	7,*197*
Actinomycins	10,*29*
Adriamycin	10,*43*
Aflatoxins	1,*145* (corr. 7,*319*)
	(corr. 8,*349*)
	10,*51*
Aldrin	5,*25*
Amaranth	8,*41*
para-Aminoazobenzene	8,*53*
ortho-Aminoazotoluene	8,*61* (corr. 11,*295*)
4-Aminobiphenyl	1,*74* (corr. 10,*343*)
2-Amino-5-(5-nitro-2-furyl)-1,3,4-thiadiazole	7,*143*
Amitrole	7,*31*
Anaesthetics, volatile	11,*285*
Aniline	4,*27* (corr. 7,*320*)
Apholate	9,*31*
Aramite^R	5,*39*
Arsenic and inorganic arsenic compounds	2,*48*
Arsenic (inorganic)	
Arsenic pentoxide	
Arsenic trioxide	
Calcium arsenate	
Calcium arsenite	
Potassium arsenate	
Potassium arsenite	
Sodium arsenate	
Sodium arsenite	
Asbestos	2,*17* (corr. 7,*319*)
Amosite	
Anthophyllite	

Chrysotile	<u>2</u>,17	
Crocidolite		
Auramine	<u>1</u>,69	(corr. <u>7</u>,319)
Azaserine	<u>10</u>,73	
Aziridine	<u>9</u>,37	
2-(1-Aziridinyl)ethanol	<u>9</u>,47	
Aziridyl benzoquinone	<u>9</u>,51	
Azobenzene	<u>8</u>,75	
Benz[c]acridine	<u>3</u>,241	
Benz[a]anthracene	<u>3</u>,45	
Benzene	<u>7</u>,203	(corr. <u>11</u>,295)
Benzidine	<u>1</u>,80	
Benzo[b]fluoranthene	<u>3</u>,69	
Benzo[j]fluoranthene	<u>3</u>,82	
Benzo[a]pyrene	<u>3</u>,91	
Benzo[e]pyrene	<u>3</u>,137	
Benzyl chloride	<u>11</u>,217	
Beryllium and beryllium compounds	<u>1</u>,17	
Beryl ore		
Beryllium oxide		
Beryllium phosphate		
Beryllium sulphate		
BHC (technical grades)	<u>5</u>,47	
Bis(1-aziridinyl)morpholinophosphine sulphide	<u>9</u>,55	
Bis(2-chloroethyl)ether	<u>9</u>,117	
N,N'-Bis(2-chloroethyl)-2-naphthylamine	<u>4</u>,119	
Bis(chloromethyl)ether	<u>4</u>,231	
1,4-Butanediol dimethanesulphonate	<u>4</u>,247	
β-Butyrolactone	<u>11</u>,225	
γ-Butyrolactone	<u>11</u>,231	
Cadmium and cadmium compounds	<u>2</u>,74	
	<u>11</u>,39	
Cadmium acetate		
Cadmium carbonate		
Cadmium chloride		

Cadmium oxide	2,74, 11,39
Cadmium powder	
Cadmium sulphate	
Cadmium sulphide	
Cantharidin	10,79
Carbon tetrachloride	1,53
Carmoisine	8,83
Chlorambucil	9,125
Chloramphenicol	10,85
Chlormadinone acetate	6,149
Chlorobenzilate	5,75
Chloroform	1,61
Chloromethyl methyl ether	4,239
Cholesterol	10,99
Chromium and inorganic chromium compounds	2,100
Barium chromate	
Calcium chromate	
Chromic chromate	
Chromic oxide	
Chromium acetate	
Chromium carbonate	
Chromium dioxide	
Chromium phosphate	
Chromium trioxide	
Lead chromate	
Potassium chromate	
Potassium dichromate	
Sodium chromate	
Sodium dichromate	
Strontium chromate	
Zinc chromate hydroxide	
Chrysene	3,159
Chrysoidine	8,91
C.I. Disperse Yellow 3	8,97
Citrus Red No. 2	8,101

Coumarin	*10*,113
Cycasin	*1*,157 (corr. *7*,319)
	10,121
Cyclochlorotine	*10*,139
Cyclophosphamide	*9*,135
Daunomycin	*10*,145
D & C Red No. 9	*8*,107
DDT and associated substances	*5*,83 (corr. 7,320)
DDD (TDE)	
DDE	
Diacetylaminoazotoluene	*8*,113
2,6-Diamino-3-(phenylazo)pyridine (hydrochloride)	*8*,117
Diazomethane	*7*,223
Dibenz[*a,h*]acridine	*3*,247
Dibenz[*a,j*]acridine	*3*,254
Dibenz[*a,h*]anthracene	*3*,178
7H-Dibenzo[*c,g*]carbazole	*3*,260
Dibenzo[*h,rst*]pentaphene	*3*,197
Dibenzo[*a,e*]pyrene	*3*,201
Dibenzo[*a,h*]pyrene	*3*,207
Dibenzo[*a,i*]pyrene	*3*,215
Dibenzo[*a,l*]pyrene	*3*,224
ortho-Dichlorobenzene	*7*,231
para-Dichlorobenzene	*7*,231
3,3'-Dichlorobenzidine	*4*,49
Dieldrin	*5*,125
Diepoxybutane	*11*,115
1,2-Diethylhydrazine	*4*,153
Diethylstilboestrol	*6*,55
Diethyl sulphate	*4*,277
Diglycidyl resorcinol ether	*11*,125
Dihydrosafrole	*1*,170
	10,233
Dimethisterone	*6*,167

3,3'-Dimethoxybenzidine (*o*-Dianisidine)	*4,41*
para-Dimethylaminoazobenzene	*8,125*
para-Dimethylaminobenzenediazo sodium sulphonate	*8,147*
trans-2[(Dimethylamino)methylimino]-5-[2-(5-nitro-2-furyl)vinyl]-1,3,4-oxadiazole	*7,147*
3,3'-Dimethylbenzidine (*o*-Tolidine)	*1,87*
1,1-Dimethylhydrazine	*4,137*
1,2-Dimethylhydrazine	*4,145* (corr. *7,320*)
Dimethyl sulphate	*4,271*
Dinitrosopentamethylenetetramine	*11,241*
1,4-Dioxane	*11,247*
Endrin	*5,157*
Epichlorohydrin	*11,131*
1-Epoxyethyl-3,4-epoxycyclohexane	*11,141*
3,4-Epoxy-6-methylcyclohexylmethyl-3,4-epoxy-6-methylcyclohexane carboxylate	*11,147*
cis-9,10-Epoxystearic acid	*11,153*
Ethinyloestradiol	*6,77*
Ethylene oxide	*11,157*
Ethylene sulphide	*11,257*
Ethylenethiourea	*7,45*
Ethyl methanesulphonate	*7,245*
Ethynodiol diacetate	*6,173*
Evans blue	*8,151*
2-(2-Formylhydrazino)-4-(5-nitro-2-furyl)thiazole	*7,151* (corr. *11,295*)
Fusarenon-X	*11,169*
Glycidaldehyde	*11,175*
Glycidyl oleate	*11,183*
Glycidyl stearate	*11,187*
Griseofulvin	*10,153*
Haematite	*1,29*
Heptachlor and its epoxide	*5,173*
Hydrazine	*4,127*
4-Hydroxyazobenzene	*8,157*
Hydroxysenkirkine	*10,265*

Indeno[1,2,3-cd]pyrene	3,229
Iron-dextran complex	2,161
Iron-dextrin complex	2,161 (corr. 7,319)
Iron oxide	1,29
Iron sorbitol-citric acid complex	2,161
Isatidine	10,269
Isonicotinic acid hydrazide	4,159
Isosafrole	1,169
Jacobine	10,275
Lasiocarpine	10,281
Lead salts	1,40 (corr. 7,319)
	(corr. 8,349)
Lead acetate	
Lead arsenate	
Lead carbonate	
Lead phosphate	
Lead subacetate	
Lindane	5,47
Luteoskyrin	10,163
Magenta	4,57 (corr. 7,320)
Maleic hydrazide	4,173
Mannomustine (dihydrochloride)	9,157
Medphalan	9,167
Medroxyprogesterone acetate	6,157
Melphalan	9,167
Merphalan	9,167
Mestranol	6,87
Methoxychlor	5,193
2-Methylaziridine	9,61
Methylazoxymethanol acetate	1,164
N-Methyl-N,4-dinitrosoaniline	1,141
4,4'-Methylene bis(2-chloroaniline)	4,65
4,4'-Methylene bis(2-methylaniline)	4,73
4,4'-Methylenedianiline	4,79 (corr. 7,320)

Methyl methanesulphonate	<u>7</u>,*253*
N-Methyl-N'-nitro-N-nitrosoguanidine	<u>4</u>,*183*
Methyl red	<u>8</u>,*161*
Methylthiouracil	<u>7</u>,*53*
Mirex	<u>5</u>,*203*
Mitomycin C	<u>10</u>,*171*
Monocrotaline	<u>10</u>,*291*
5-(Morpholinomethyl)-3-[(5-nitrofurfurylidene)amino]-2-oxazolidinone	<u>7</u>,*161*
Mustard gas	<u>9</u>,*181*
1-Naphthylamine	<u>4</u>,*87* (corr. <u>8</u>,*349*)
2-Naphthylamine	<u>4</u>,*97*
Native carrageenans	<u>10</u>,*181* (corr. <u>11</u>,*295*)
Nickel and nickel compounds	<u>2</u>,*126* (corr. <u>7</u>,*319*)
	<u>11</u>,*75*
Nickel acetate	
Nickel carbonate	
Nickel carbonyl	
Nickelocene	
Nickel oxide	
Nickel powder	
Nickel subsulphide	
Nickel sulphate	
4-Nitrobiphenyl	<u>4</u>,*113*
5-Nitro-2-furaldehyde semicarbazone	<u>7</u>,*171*
1[(5-Nitrofurfurylidene)amino]-2-imidazolidinone	<u>7</u>,*181*
N-[4-(5-Nitro-2-furyl)-2-thiazolyl]acetamide	<u>1</u>,*181*
	<u>7</u>,*185*
Nitrogen mustard (hydrochloride)	<u>9</u>,*193*
Nitrogen mustard N-oxide (hydrochloride)	<u>9</u>,*209*
N-Nitroso-di-n-butylamine	<u>4</u>,*197*
N-Nitrosodiethylamine	<u>1</u>,*107* (corr. <u>11</u>,*295*)
N-Nitrosodimethylamine	<u>1</u>,*95*
Nitrosoethylurea	<u>1</u>,*135*
Nitrosomethylurea	<u>1</u>,*125*

N-Nitroso-N-methylurethane	4,*211*
Norethisterone	6,*179*
Norethisterone acetate	6,*179*
Norethynodrel	6,*191*
Norgestrel	6,*201*
Ochratoxin A	10,*191*
Oestradiol-17β	6,*99*
Oestradiol mustard	9,*217*
Oestriol	6,*117*
Oestrone	6,*123*
Oil orange SS	8,*165*
Orange I	8,*173*
Orange G	8,*181*
Parasorbic acid	10,*199*
Patulin	10,*205*
Penicillic acid	10,*211*
Phenoxybenzamine (hydrochloride)	9,*223*
Polychlorinated biphenyls	7,*261*
Ponceau MX	8,*189*
Ponceau 3R	8,*199*
Ponceau SX	8,*207*
Progesterone	6,*135*
1,3-Propane sultone	4,*253*
β-Propiolactone	4,*259*
Propylene oxide	11,*191*
Propylthiouracil	7,*67*
Quintozene (Pentachloronitrobenzene)	5,*211*
Reserpine	10,*217*
Retrorsine	10,*303*
Riddelliine	10,*313*
Saccharated iron oxide	2,*161*
Safrole	1,*169*
	10,*231*
Scarlet red	8,*217*
Selenium and selenium compounds	9,*245*

Senecipylline	10,*319*
Senkirkine	10,*327*
Soot, tars and shale oils	3,*22*
Sterigmatocystin	1,*175*
	10,*245*
Streptozotocin	4,*221*
Styrene oxide	11,*201*
Sudan I	8,*225*
Sudan II	8,*233*
Sudan III	8,*241*
Sudan brown RR	8,*249*
Sudan red 7B	8,*253*
Sunset yellow FCF	8,*257*
Tannic acid	10,*253*
Tannins	10,*254*
Terpene polychlorinates (Strobane[R])	5,*219*
Testosterone	6,*209*
Tetraethyllead	2,*150*
Tetramethyllead	2,*150*
Thioacetamide	7,*77*
Thiouracil	7,*85*
Thiourea	7,*95*
Trichloroethylene	11,*263*
Trichlorotriethylamine hydrochloride	9,*229*
Triethylene glycol diglycidyl ether	11,*209*
Tris(aziridinyl)-*para*-benzoquinone	9,*67*
Tris(1-aziridinyl)phosphine oxide	9,*75*
Tris(1-aziridinyl)phosphine sulphide	9,*85*
2,4,6-Tris(1-aziridinyl)-*s*-triazine	9,*95*
Tris(2-methyl-1-aziridinyl)phosphine oxide	9,*107*
Trypan blue	8,*267*
Uracil mustard	9,*235*
Urethane	7,*111*
Vinyl chloride	7,*291*
4-Vinylcyclohexene	11,*277*

Yellow AB	8,279
Yellow OB	8,287

www.ingramcontent.com/pod-product-compliance
Ingram Content Group UK Ltd.
Pitfield, Milton Keynes, MK11 3LW, UK
UKHW051259180426
11947UKWH00020B/1790